# DEMENTIA

## A PUBLIC HEALTH PRIORITY

Alzheimer's Disease International

World Health Organization

**WHO Library Cataloguing-in-Publication Data:**

Dementia: a public health priority.

1. Aging – psychology. 2. Dementia – epidemiology. 3. Dementia – prevention and control. 4. Caregivers – psychology. 5. Health services for the aged – economics. 6. Long-term care. 7. Health priorities. I. World Health Organization.

ISBN 978 92 4 156445 8
(NLM classification: WM 200)



Printed in United Kingdom

# CONTENTS

# FOREWORD

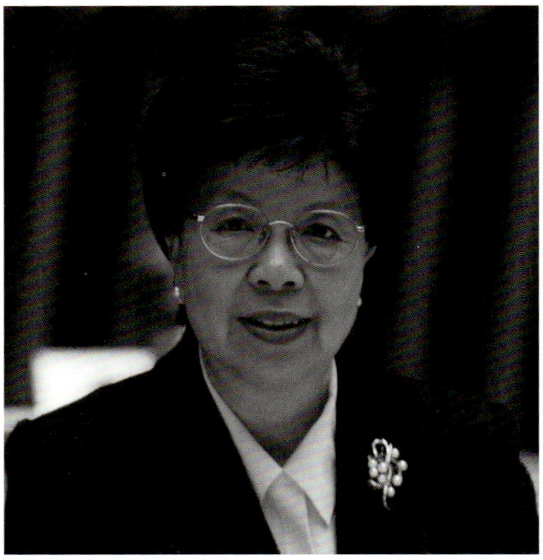

The world's population is ageing. Improvements in health care in the past century have contributed to people living longer and healthier lives. However, this has also resulted in an increase in the number of people with non-communicable diseases, including dementia. Current estimates indicate 35.6 million people worldwide are living with dementia. This number will double by 2030 and more than triple by 2050. Dementia doesn't just affect individuals. It also affects and changes the lives of family members. Dementia is a costly condition in its social, economic, and health dimensions. Nearly 60 percent of the burden of dementia is concentrated in low- and middle-income countries and this is likely to increase in coming years.

The need for long-term care for people with dementia strains health and social systems, and budgets. The catastrophic cost of care drives millions of households below the poverty line. The overwhelming number of people whose lives are altered by dementia, combined with the staggering economic burden on families and nations, makes dementia a public health priority. The cost of caring for people with dementia is likely to rise even faster than its prevalence, and thus it is important that societies are prepared to address the social and economic burden caused by dementia.

In 2008, WHO launched the Mental Health Gap Action Programme (mhGAP), which included dementia as a priority condition. In 2011, the High-level Meeting of the United Nations General Assembly on prevention and control of non-communicable diseases adopted a Political Declaration that acknowledged that "the global burden and threat of non-communicable diseases constitutes one of the major challenges for development in the twenty-first century" and recognized that "mental and neurological disorders, including Alzheimer's disease, are an important cause of morbidity and contribute to the global non-communicable disease burden."

It is against this background that I am pleased to present the report, "Dementia: a public health priority." This report makes a major contribution to our understanding of dementia and its impact on individuals, families, and society. I would like to thank the representative organizations of people with dementia and their caregivers, who have greatly enriched both the scope of the report and its value as a practical tool.

The report provides the knowledge base for a global and national response to facilitate governments, policy-makers, and other stakeholders to address the impact of dementia as an increasing threat to global health. I call upon all stakeholders to make health and social care systems informed and responsive to this impending threat.

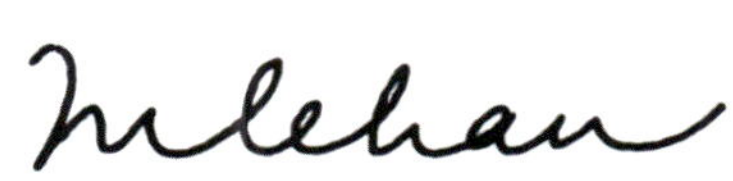

Dr Margaret Chan

Director-General
World Health Organization

# PREFACE

Dementia is seriously disabling for those who have it and is often devastating for their caregivers and families. With an increasing number of people being affected by dementia, almost everyone knows someone who has dementia or whose life has been touched by it. The number of people living with dementia worldwide is currently estimated at 35.6 million. This number will double by 2030 and more than triple by 2050.

The high global prevalence, economic impact of dementia on families, caregivers and communities, and the associated stigma and social exclusion present a significant public health challenge. The global health community has recognized the need for action and to place dementia on the public health agenda.

The World Health Organization and Alzheimer's Disease International, an international NGO in official relations with WHO, jointly developed the report, *Dementia: a public health priority.* The purpose of this report is to raise awareness of dementia as a public health priority, to articulate a public health approach and to advocate for action at international and national levels based on the principles of evidence, equity, inclusion and integration.

The report aims to encourage country preparedness by strengthening or developing policy and implementing it through plans and programmes which enhance dementia care in order to improve the social well-being and quality of life of those living with dementia and their caregivers. The reports includes an overview of global epidemiology and the impact of dementia, national-level approaches to dementia including the role of health and social care systems and workforce, issues around caregiving and caregivers, and awareness raising and advocacy for dementia.

As this would not have been possible without the significant contribution of representative organizations of people with dementia and their caregivers, we would like to thank them for their invaluable work and support.

The report is expected to be a resource that will facilitate governments, policy-makers, and other stakeholders to address the impact of dementia as an increasing threat to global health. It is hoped that the key messages in the report will promote dementia as a public health and social care priority worldwide.

Dr Shekhar Saxena
Director, Department of Mental Health and Substance Abuse
World Health Organization

Mr Marc Wortmann
Executive Director
Alzheimer's Disease International

# ABBREVIATIONS

| | |
|---|---|
| A&TSI | Aboriginal and Torres Strait Islander |
| ADI | Alzheimer's Disease International |
| ADL | Activities of daily living |
| AIDS | Acquired Immunodeficiency Syndrome |
| APOE | Apolipoprotein E |
| CI | Confidence interval |
| CRPD | Convention on the Rights of Persons with Disabilities |
| CSAP | Carer's Strategy and Action Plan |
| DLB | Dementia with Lewy bodies |
| DSM | Diagnostic and Statistical Manual of Mental Disorders |
| EuroCoDe | European Collaboration on Dementia |
| EURODEM | European Community Concerted Action on the Epidemiology and Prevention of Dementia |
| FTD | Frontotemporal dementia |
| GBD | Global burden of disease |
| GDP | Gross domestic product |
| HAART | Highly Active Antiretroviral Therapy |
| HAND | HIV-associated neurocognitive disorder |
| HHS | Health and Human Services |
| HIV | Human Immunodeficiency Virus |
| HR | Hazard ratio |
| IADL | Instrumental activities of daily living |
| ICD | International Statistical Classification of Diseases and Related Health Problems |
| IMPACT | Important Perspectives on Alzheimer's Care and Treatment |
| LMIC | Low- and middle-income countries |
| MAIA | Maisons pour l'Autonomie et Intégration des malades Alzheimer |
| mhGAP | Mental Health Gap Action Programme |
| MNS | Mental, neurological and substance use |
| NIH | National Institutes of Health |
| OECD | Organisation for Economic Co-operation and Development |
| PAR | Population attributable risk |
| PPP | Purchasing power parity |
| REACH | Resources for Enhancing Alzheimer's Caregiver Health |
| RR | Relative risk |
| SEK | Swedish krona |
| VaD | Vascular dementia |
| WHO | World Health Organization |
| YOD | Young onset dementia |

# ACKNOWLEDGEMENTS


## CONCEPTUALIZATION AND GUIDANCE

Shekhar Saxena (WHO), Marc Wortmann (UK), Daisy Acosta (Dominican Republic), Martin Prince (UK), Ennapadam. S Krishnamoorthy (India).

## PROJECT COORDINATION AND EDITING

Tarun Dua (WHO), Pamela Nichols (Australia), Yutaro Setoya (WHO).

## TECHNICAL CONTRIBUTION AND REVIEW

### WORKING GROUP MEMBERS

**Working Group 1:** *Epidemiology, types, classification and cost.* Steve T. DeKosky (USA), Lutz Frölich (Germany), Miia Kivipelto (Sweden), Martin Prince (Chair, UK), Anders Wimo (Sweden).

**Working Group 2:** *Policy, legislation, health care system and social support structure.* Daisy Acosta (Chair, Dominican Republic), Marco Blom (Netherlands), Panteleimon Giannakopoulos (Switzerland), Oye Gureje (Nigeria), Peter Lloyd-Sherlock (UK), Glenn Rees (Australia), Michael Splaine (USA).

**Working Group 3:** *Awareness raising and education, public and professional attitudes and ethical aspects.* Sabine Bährer-Kohler (Switzerland), Murna Downs (UK), Mariella Guerra (Peru), Tony Hope (UK), Diane Mansour (Lebanon), Mary Marshall (UK), Myrra Vernooij-Dassen (Netherlands), Marc Wortmann (Chair, UK).

**Working Group 4:** *Caregivers.* Stefanie Auer (Austria), Henry Brodaty (Australia), Dolores Gallagher-Thompson (Canada), Iva Holmerova (Czech Republic), Mira Josic de Hernandez (Venezuela), Ennapadam S. Krishnamoorthy (Chair, India), Yoshio Miyake (Japan), Ameenah Sorefan (Mauritius), Richard Uwakwe (Nigeria).

### INTERNATIONAL CONTRIBUTORS

Happy Kokou Agoudavi (Togo), Sally-Marie Bamford (UK), Sube Banerjee (UK), Matthew Baumgart (USA), Pierre-Emmanuel Brugeron (France), Venessa Curnow (Australia), Hidetoshi Endo (Japan), Maree Farrow (Australia), Giovanni B. Frisoni (Italy), Saad Ghalib (United Arab Emirates), Kentaro Horibe (Japan), Georges E. Karam (Lebanon), Sujaya Krishnan (India), Sunghee Lee (Republic of Korea), Sandrine Lemery (France), Florence Lustman (France), Diane Mansour (Lebanon), Urs P. Mosimann (Switzerland), Flavio Paoletti (Italy), Yasmin Raashid (Pakistan), Perminder S. Sachdev (Australia), Linda Seaward (UK), Ana Luisa Sosa Ortiz (Mexico), Jotheeswaran Thiyagarajan (India), Babu Varghese (India), Huali Wang (China).

### EXPERT REVIEWERS

Ricardo F. Allegri (Argentina), Nana Araba Apt (Ghana), Takashi Asada (Japan), Nelleen Baboolal (Trinidad and Tobago), Paulo Caramelli (Brazil), Monique Chaaya (Lebanon), Ding Ding (China), S. K. Das (India), Patricio Fuentes (Chile), Yueqin Huang (China), Steve Iliffe (UK), John Joska (South Africa), Ichiro Kai (Japan), Norito Kawakami (Japan), Katsunori Kondo (Japan), Facundo Manes (Argentina), Walter Mangezi (Zimbabwe), Kozo Matsubayashi (Japan), Ana Claire Meyer (USA), Ndahambelela Mthoko (Namibia), Sekai Nhiwatiwa (Zimbabwe), Adesola Ogunniyi (Nigeria), Toshiyuki Ojima (Japan), Corinna Porteri (Italy), Pierre-Marie Preux (France), Vorapun Senanarong (Thailand), Richard Schultz (Canada), K. S. Shaji (India), William Thies (USA), Johan Vos (New Zealand), Bengt Winblad (Sweden).

### SURVEY RESPONDENTS

Happy Kokou Agoudavi (Togo), Ana Baldoni (Argentina), Debbie Benczkowski (Canada), Md Shahjahan Biswas (Bangladesh), Nora Eneyda de la Garza-Acevedo (Mexico), Scott Dudgeon (Canada), Faraneh Farin (Iran), Patricio Fuentes (Chile), Maria Gantman (Russian Federation), Saad Ghalib (United Arab Emirates), Mariella Guerra (Peru), Dagoberto Guilamo (Dominican Republic), Azizul Haque (Bangladesh), Hasmet A. Hanagasi (Turkey), Agus Hartanto (Indonesia), Heike Hesse (Honduras), Arsenio Hueros (Spain), Jeremy Hughes (UK), Lidia Iriarte (Argentina), Hussain Jafri (Pakistan), Sabine Jansen (Germany), Thierry Jarlet (France), Mira Josic de Hernandez (Venezuela), Ong Eng Joo (Malaysia), Martina Kane (UK), Yim Khai Kee (Malaysia), Fugen Kural (Turkey), Sunghee Lee (Republic of Korea), Diane Mansour (Lebanon), Birgitta Martensson (Switzerland), Yoko Mizutani (Japan), Martina WS Nasrun (Indonesia), David Ndetei (Kenya), Glenn Rees (Australia), Jesús Rodrigo (Spain), Jacob Roy (India), Alicja Sadowska (Poland), Tami Tamitegama (Sri Lanka), Richard Uwakwe (Nigeria), Yin-Hua Wang (China), Huali Wang (China), Mirka Wojciechowska (Poland), Ryu Yoshino (Japan).

### WHO HEADQUARTERS

Katerina Ainali, John Beard, Nicolas Clark, Dan Chisholm, Natalie Drew, Alexandra Fleischmann, Daniela Fuhr, Michelle Funk, Colin Mathers, Jodi Morris, Vladimir Poznyak, Geoffrey Reed, Andreas Reis, Dag Rekve, Chiara Servili, Thomas Shakespeare, Sarah Skeen, Kanna Sugiura, Mark van Ommeren, Isy Vromans, Taghi M. Yasamy.

### WHO REGIONAL OFFICES

Sebastiana Da Gama Nkomo & Carina Ferreira-Borges, WHO Regional Office for Africa; Jorge Rodriguez, WHO Regional Office for the Americas; Vijay Chandra, WHO Regional Office for South-East Asia; Matthijs Muijen, WHO Regional Office for Europe; Khalid Saeed, WHO Regional Office for the Eastern Mediterranean; Xiangdong Wang, WHO Regional Office for the Western Pacific.

### INTERNS

Mika Mizunuma, Keiko Sakurai.

## ADMINISTRATIVE SUPPORT

Adeline Loo (WHO), Grazia Motturi (WHO), Sarah Smith (UK), Rosemary Westermeyer (WHO).

## PRODUCTION TEAM

**Editing:** David Bramley, Switzerland
**Graphic design and layout:** Erica Lefstad and Christian Bäuerle, Germany

## PHOTOS

**Cover page** (by Cathy Greenblat)
Bhanumathi brushing away the evil spirits from an aide – Bangalore, India
**Executive summary** (by Cathy Greenblat)
A Japanese woman at a group home in Kyoto peacefully admires the bamboo garden – Kyoto, Japan
**Chapter 1 Introduction** (by Cathy Greenblat)
Melissa, the daughter of a staff member, is completely comfortable with residents of the Silverado Senior Living residential community who give her many signs of affection – Escondido, California
**Chapter 2 Epidemiology of dementia** (by Alzheimer's Disease International)
An interview being conducted for the Indianapolis-Ibadan Dementia Project – Ibadan, Nigeria
**Chapter 3 Dementia policy and plans** (by Leonardo Ramírez)
Yolanda and Jose on his birthday. Jose is responsible for all the care of Yolanda and doesn't accept the help of others. He says that when he married her, he swore to love and care for her in any adversity – Caracas, Venezuela
**Chapter 4 Dementia health and social care systems** (by Cathy Greenblat)
Arthur joined six fellow residents on a Fourth of July outing and had a good time. The next day he napped peacefully in the salon – Escondido, California
**Chapter 5 Dementia caregiving and caregivers** (by Cathy Greenblat)
Carole and her mother, MaryLou, holding hands the day before MaryLou died – Escondido, California
**Chapter 6 Public understanding of dementia** (by Cathy Greenblat)
Despite Lars' weakened condition, he was happy to hold the hand of Heather, the music therapist, while she played the guitar and to sing with her – Escondido, California
**Chapter 7 The way forward** (by Cathy Greenblat)
Meredith likes to look elegant and sporty every day and she was one of the first to be seated at the July 4th party – Escondido, California

*WHO would like to thank Alzheimer's Disease International (ADI), UK; Centre collaborateur de l'OMS pour la Psychiatrie de la Personne âgée, Service Universitaire de Psychiatrie de l'Age Avancé (SUPAA) Lausanne, Switzerland; Centre collaborateur de l'OMS pour la Recherche et la Formation en Santé mentale, Université de Genève, Geneva, Switzerland, for their contributions.*

*ADI would like to thank Alzheimer's Australia, Alzheimer's Australia (West Australia), MetLife Foundation, Stichting Alzheimer Nederland, and Vradenburg Foundation, for their contributions.*

# EXECUTIVE SUMMARY

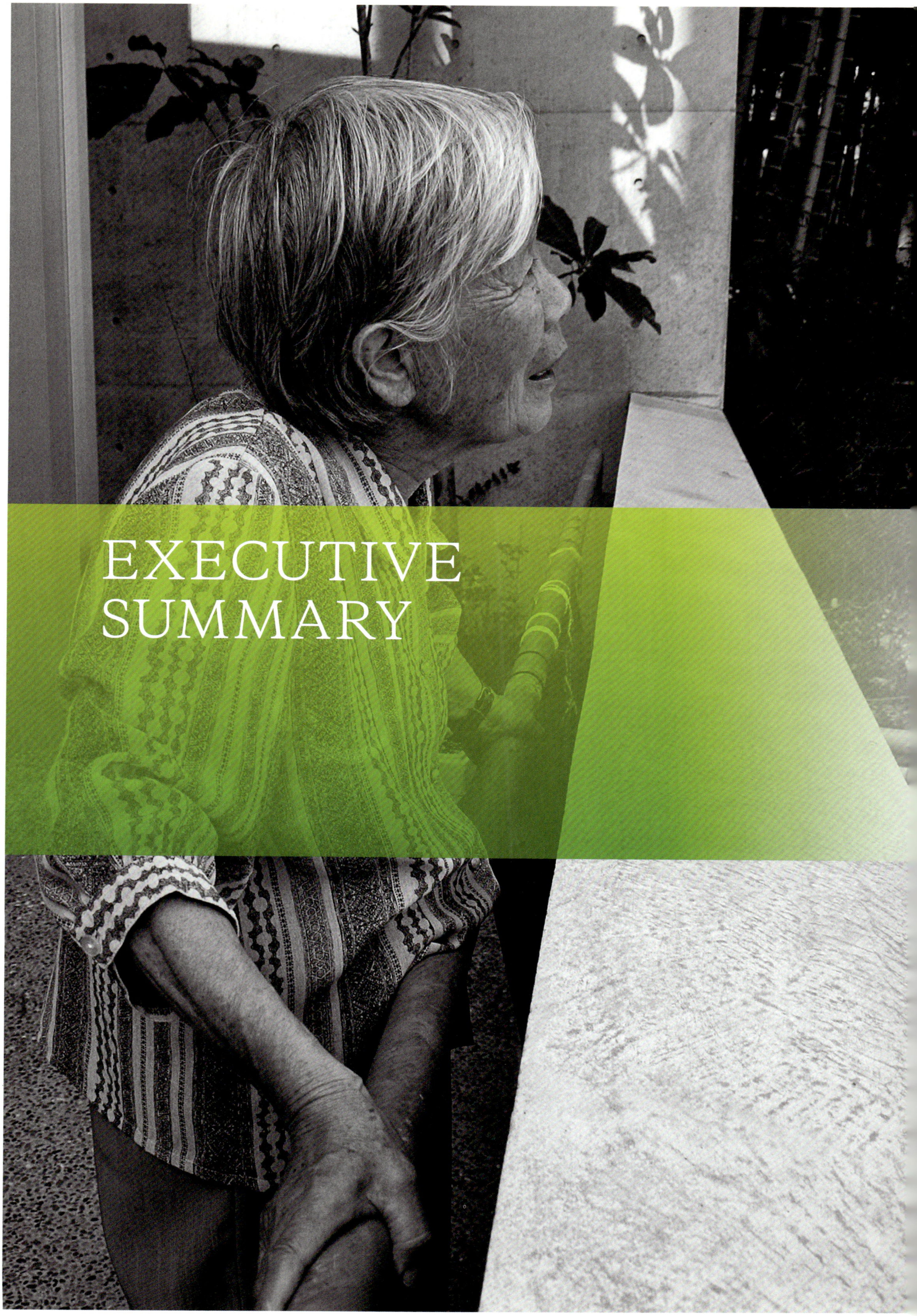

The world's population is ageing. Improvements in health care in the past century have contributed to people living longer and healthier lives. However, this has also resulted in an increase in the number of people with noncommunicable diseases, including dementia. Although dementia mainly affects older people, it is not a normal part of ageing. Dementia is a syndrome, usually of a chronic or progressive nature, caused by a variety of brain illnesses that affect memory, thinking, behaviour and ability to perform everyday activities.

Dementia is overwhelming not only for the people who have it, but also for their caregivers and families. It is one of the major causes of disability and dependency among older people worldwide. There is lack of awareness and understanding of dementia, at some level, in most countries, resulting in stigmatization, barriers to diagnosis and care, and impacting caregivers, families and societies physically, psychologically and economically. Dementia can no longer be neglected but should be considered a part of the public health agenda in all countries.

The objective of this report is to raise awareness of dementia as a public health priority, to articulate a public health approach and to advocate for action at international and national levels based on the principles of inclusion, integration, equity and evidence.

## BURDEN OF DEMENTIA

We have a growing body of evidence on the global prevalence and incidence of dementia, the associated mortality and the global economic cost. Most of the information is from high-income countries with some data becoming increasingly available from low- and middle-income countries (LMIC).

Prevalence and incidence projections indicate that the number of people with dementia will continue to grow, particularly among the oldest old, and countries in demographic transition will experience the greatest growth. The total number of people with dementia worldwide in 2010 is estimated at 35.6 million and is projected to nearly double every 20 years, to 65.7 million in 2030 and 115.4 million in 2050. The total number of new cases of dementia each year worldwide is nearly 7.7 million, implying one new case every four seconds.

The total estimated worldwide costs of dementia were US$ 604 billion in 2010. In high-income countries, informal care (45%) and formal social care (40%) account for the majority of costs, while the proportionate contribution of direct medical costs (15%) is much lower. In low-income and lower-middle-income countries direct social care costs are small, and informal care costs (i.e. unpaid care provided by the family) predominate. Changing population demographics in many LMIC may lead to a decline in the ready availability of extended family members in the coming decades.

Research identifying modifiable risk factors of dementia is in its infancy. In the meantime, primary prevention should focus on targets suggested by current evidence. These include countering risk factors for vascular disease, including diabetes, midlife hypertension, midlife obesity, smoking, and physical inactivity.

## COUNTRY PREPAREDNESS FOR DEMENTIA

The challenges to governments to respond to the growing numbers of people with dementia are substantial. A broad public health approach is needed to improve the care and quality of life of people with dementia and family caregivers. The aims and objectives of the approach should either be articulated in a stand-alone dementia policy or plan or be integrated into existing health, mental health or old-age policies and plans. Some high-income countries have launched policies, plans, strategies or frameworks to respond to the impact of dementia.

There are several key issues that are common to many national dementia policies and plans, and these may be necessary to ensure that needs are addressed in an effective and sustainable manner. These include: scoping the problem; involving all the relevant stakeholders, including civil society groups; identifying priority areas for action; implementing the policy and plan; committing resources; having intersectoral collaboration; developing a time frame; and monitoring and evaluation.

The priority areas of action that need to be addressed within the policy and plan include raising awareness, timely diagnosis, commitment to good quality continuing care and services, caregiver support, workforce training, prevention and research.

People with dementia and their families face significant financial impact from the cost of providing health and social care and from reduction or loss of income. Universal social support through pensions and insurance schemes could provide protection to this vulnerable group.

Formal recognition of the rights of people with dementia and their caregivers through legislation and regulatory processes will help reduce discriminatory practices. Fundamental to upholding a person's rights is the recognition of capacity in persons with dementia. Where capacity is impaired due to dementia, legal provisions should recognize and protect the right to appropriate autonomy and self-determination including substitute or supported decision-making and procedures for implementing advance directives. Education and support relating to ethical decision-making and human rights should be an essential part of capacity-building for all involved in providing dementia care, including policy-makers, professionals and families.

## HEALTH AND SOCIAL SYSTEMS DEVELOPMENT

The health and social care needs of the large and rapidly growing numbers of frail dependent older persons should be a matter of great concern for policy-makers in all countries. This is particularly so for LMIC which will experience the greatest increase in ageing in the coming decades.

This challenges governments to develop and improve services for people with dementia, focusing on earlier diagnosis, provision of support in the community, and a responsive health and social care sector. Integrated and coordinated health and social pathways and services will be needed to cater for the changing needs of people with dementia and their caregivers. Such pathways should ensure that the needs of specific or minority population groups are taken into account.

Improved community support will assist families to provide care for longer and to delay or reduce reliance on high-cost residential care. Where resources are finite, especially in LMIC, a focus on community outreach could be an efficient use of scarce resources to improve the quality of life of people with dementia and their caregivers. The effectiveness of task shifting (with appropriate guidelines and training) in LMIC should be further evaluated as a solution to the under-supply of a professional workforce.

Capacity-building of the workforce is essential to improve knowledge and awareness of the benefits of a coordinated response to care. Dementia care, long-term care and chronic disease management incorporating a multidisciplinary team should form part of professional education and should be supported by the development of appropriate practice guidelines. In a world with an increasingly mobile population, the migrant workforce brings its own set of challenges that need to be understood and addressed.

## SUPPORT FOR INFORMAL CARE AND CAREGIVERS

Dementia has an immense impact on the lives of the family, and particularly the person who takes the primary role in providing care. Most care is provided by family and other informal support systems in the community and most caregivers are women. However, changing population demographics may reduce the availability of informal caregivers in the future.

The provision of care to a person with dementia can result in significant strain for those who provide most of that care. The stressors are physical, emotional and economic. A range of programmes and services have been developed in high-income countries to assist family caregivers and to reduce strain. The beneficial effects of caregiver interventions in decreasing the institutionalization of the care recipient have been clearly demonstrated.

Evidence from LMIC also suggests that home-based support for caregivers of persons with dementia, emphasizing the use of locally-available low-cost human resources, is feasible, acceptable and leads to significant improvements in caregiver mental health and in the burden of caring. Despite evidence of effectiveness, there have been no successful examples of scale-up in any of the health systems in which the evaluative research has been conducted. Further research should focus on implementation in order to inform the process of scale-up.

Despite the availability of services in some countries or parts of countries, there are barriers to uptake. Lack of awareness of services, lack of understanding or stigma attached to the syndrome, previous poor experience with services, and cultural, language and financial barriers creates obstacles to service utilization. Information and education campaigns for the public – including people with dementia, their caregivers and families – can improve service utilization by raising awareness, improving understanding and decreasing stigmatizing attitudes.

Support is needed to enable informal caregivers to be able to continue in their role for as long as possible. Support includes information to aid understanding, skills to assist in caring, respite to enable engagement in other activities, and financial support.

## AWARENESS-RAISING AND ADVOCACY

Despite the growing impact globally, a lack of understanding of dementia contributes to fears and to stigmatization. For those who are living with dementia (both the person and their family), the stigma contributes to social isolation and to delays in seeking diagnosis and help.

There is an urgent need to improve the awareness and understanding of dementia across all levels of society as a step towards improving the quality of life of people with dementia and their caregivers. Governments have a role to play in resourcing public awareness campaigns and in ensuring that key stakeholders are involved in such campaigns.

Awareness-raising campaigns should be relevant to the context and audience. They should be accurate, effective and informative and should be developed in consultation with people with dementia, their families and other stakeholders, including civil society.

## THE WAY FORWARD

The findings of this report demonstrate that dementia is a global public health challenge. A range of actions is required to improve care and services for people with dementia and their caregivers. These actions include advocacy and awareness-raising, developing and implementing dementia policies and plans, health system strengthening, capacity-building, supporting caregivers and research. The actions need to be context-specific and culturally relevant.

## KEY MESSAGES

- Dementia is not a normal part of ageing.
- 35.6 million people were estimated to be living with dementia in 2010. There are 7.7 million new cases of dementia each year, implying that there is a new case of dementia somewhere in the world every four seconds. The accelerating rates of dementia are cause for immediate action, especially in LMIC where resources are few.
- The huge cost of the disease will challenge health systems to deal with the predicted future increase of prevalence. The costs are estimated at US$ 604 billion per year at present and are set to increase even more quickly than the prevalence.
- People live for many years after the onset of symptoms of dementia. With appropriate support, many can and should be enabled to continue to engage and contribute within society and have a good quality of life.
- Dementia is overwhelming for the caregivers and adequate support is required for them from the health, social, financial and legal systems.
- Countries must include dementia on their public health agendas. Sustained action and coordination is required across multiple levels and with all stakeholders – at international, national, regional and local levels.
- People with dementia and their caregivers often have unique insights to their condition and life. They should be involved in formulating the policies, plans, laws and services that relate to them.
- The time to act is now by:
  - promoting a dementia friendly society globally;
  - making dementia a national public health and social care priority worldwide;
  - improving public and professional attitudes to, and understanding of, dementia;
  - investing in health and social systems to improve care and services for people with dementia and their caregivers;
  - increasing the priority given to dementia in the public health research agenda.

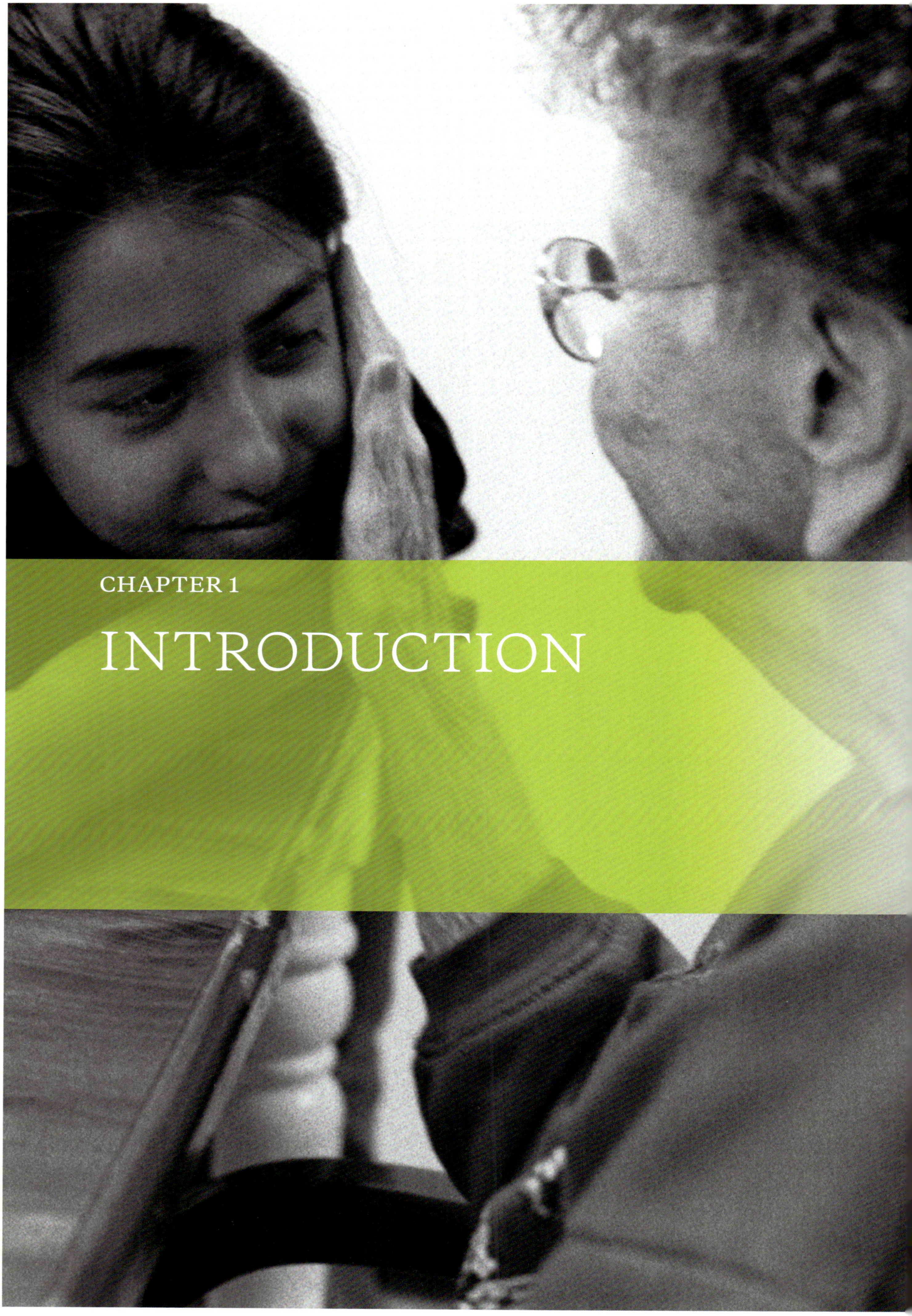

CHAPTER 1

# INTRODUCTION

## "…ALZHEIMER'S DISEASE BURDENS AN INCREASING NUMBER OF OUR NATION'S ELDERS AND THEIR FAMILIES, AND IT IS ESSENTIAL THAT WE CONFRONT THE CHALLENGE IT POSES TO OUR PUBLIC HEALTH…"

President Barack Obama, United States of America, 2011 *(1)*

Dementia is devastating not only for those persons who have it, but also for their caregivers and families. With an increasing number of people being affected by dementia, almost everyone knows someone who has dementia or whose life has been touched by it. The consequences for societies and economies are devastating everywhere, in high-income countries and low- and middle-income countries (LMIC) alike.

Although awareness of dementia as a public health issue is increasing in some high-income countries, dementia has been absent from, or low on, the health agenda of LMIC and has been minimally represented in global health efforts. This is despite the high global prevalence and economic impact of dementia on families, caregivers and communities, and the associated stigma and social exclusion.

BOX 1.1

## WHAT IS DEMENTIA?

Dementia is a syndrome due to disease of the brain – usually of a chronic or progressive nature – in which there is disturbance of multiple higher cortical functions, including memory, thinking, orientation, comprehension, calculation, learning capacity, language, and judgement. Consciousness is not clouded. The impairments of cognitive function are commonly accompanied, and occasionally preceded, by deterioration in emotional control, social behaviour, or motivation. This syndrome occurs in a large number of conditions primarily or secondarily affecting the brain *(2)*.

Alzheimer's disease is the most common form of dementia and possibly contributes to 60–70% of cases. Other major contributors include vascular dementia, dementia with Lewy bodies, and a group of diseases that contribute to frontotemporal dementia. The boundaries between subtypes are indistinct and mixed forms often co-exist *(3)*.

Dementia affects each person in a different way, depending upon the impact of the disease and the person's pre-morbid personality. The problems linked to dementia can be understood in three stages:

- early stage – first year or two;
- middle stage – second to fourth or fifth years;
- late stage – fifth year and after.

These periods are given as an approximate guideline only – sometimes people may deteriorate more quickly, sometimes more slowly. It should be noted that not all persons with dementia will display all the symptoms *(4)*.

### COMMON SYMPTOMS EXPERIENCED BY PEOPLE WITH DEMENTIA SYNDROME

| Early stage | Middle stage | Late stage |
|---|---|---|
| The early stage is often overlooked. Relatives and friends (and sometimes professionals as well) see it as "old age", just a normal part of ageing process. Because the onset of the disease is gradual, it is difficult to be sure exactly when it begins.<br>• Become forgetful, especially regarding things that just happened<br>• May have some difficulty with communication, such as difficulty in finding words<br>• Become lost in familiar places<br>• Lose track of the time, including time of day, month, year, season<br>• Have difficulty making decisions and handling personal finances<br>• Have difficulty carrying out complex household tasks<br>• Mood and behaviour:<br>– may become less active and motivated and lose interest in activities and hobbies<br>– may show mood changes, including depression or anxiety<br>– may react unusually angrily or aggressively on occasion | As the disease progresses, limitations become clearer and more restricting.<br>• Become very forgetful, especially of recent events and people's names<br>• Have difficulty comprehending time, date, place and events; may become lost at home as well as in the community<br>• Have increasing difficulty with communication (speech and comprehension)<br>• Need help with personal care (i.e. toileting, washing, dressing)<br>• Unable to successfully prepare food, cook, clean or shop<br>• Unable to live alone safely without considerable support<br>• Behaviour changes may include wandering, repeated questioning, calling out, clinging, disturbed sleeping, hallucinations (seeing or hearing things which are not there)<br>• May display inappropriate behaviour in the home or in the community (e.g. disinhibition, aggression) | The last stage is one of nearly total dependence and inactivity. Memory disturbances are very serious and the physical side of the disease becomes more obvious.<br>• Usually unaware of time and place<br>• Have difficulty understanding what is happening around them<br>• Unable to recognize relatives, friends and familiar objects<br>• Unable to eat without assistance, may have difficulty in swallowing<br>• Increasing need for assisted self-care (bathing and toileting)<br>• May have bladder and bowel incontinence<br>• Change in mobility, may be unable to walk or be confined to a wheelchair or bed<br>• Behaviour changes, may escalate and include aggression towards carer, nonverbal agitation (kicking, hitting, screaming or moaning)<br>• Unable to find his or her way around in the home |

*Source: References 3, 4.*

## DEMENTIA: A PUBLIC HEALTH ISSUE

It is estimated that by 2050 the world population over the age of 60 will be 2 billion (Figure 1.1) *(5)*. Population ageing is occurring rapidly in LMIC. A clearly negative effect of rapid ageing of the population is the increase in the number of people with dementia. Although dementia mainly affects older people, it is not a normal part of ageing.

According to different estimates, between 2% and 10% of all cases of dementia start before the age of 65. The prevalence doubles with every five-year increment in age after 65. The number of people globally who are living with dementia in 2011 is estimated to be 35.6 million, and epidemiological studies indicate that this number is expected to grow at an alarming rate. It is estimated that numbers will nearly double every 20 years, to 65.7 million in 2030 and 115.4 million in 2050 *(3)*. The majority of these people will be living in LMIC.

Dementia is one of the major causes of disability in later life. It accounts for 11.9% of the years lived with disability due to a non-communicable disease *(6)*. It is the leading cause of dependency (i.e. need for care) and disability among older persons in both high-income countries and LMIC. The estimated worldwide cost of dementia is estimated to have been US$ 604 billion in 2010. Direct medical care costs contribute to just 16% of the global cost. In low-income countries, most costs are due to informal care (i.e. unpaid care provided by family members and others) *(7)*.

While the numbers and the costs are daunting, the impact on those with the illness and on their caregivers and families is extreme – medically, psychologically and emotionally. The behavioural and psychological symptoms linked to dementia profoundly affect the quality of life of people with dementia and their caregivers.

There is a lack of awareness and understanding of dementia, at some level, in most countries. It is often considered to be a normal part of ageing or a condition for which nothing can be done. This affects people with dementia, their caregivers and families, and their support structure in a number of ways. Low awareness levels contribute to stigmatization and isolation. Poor understanding creates barriers to timely diagnosis and to accessing ongoing medical and social care, leading to a large gap in treatment.

Lack of awareness also takes its toll of the resilience of the family unit and increases financial and legal vulnerability. In many countries, including those in economic transition, the members of the extended family, who may have been able to absorb the impact of caring across the family network in the past, now live far from their kin for economic reasons. This change is likely to result in an increase in the need for formal care in coming years. At national level, the lack of awareness and lack of infrastructure for providing timely and appropriate support early in the course of the disease increase the likelihood of high costs of supporting increased dependence and morbidity.

No treatments are currently available to cure or even alter the progressive course of dementia, although numerous new therapies are being investigated in various stages of clinical trials. There is, however, much that can be offered to support and improve the lives of people with dementia and their caregivers and families. The principal goals for dementia care are:

- early diagnosis;
- optimising physical health, cognition, activity and well-being;
- detecting and treating behavioural and psychological symptoms;
- providing information and long-term support to caregivers.

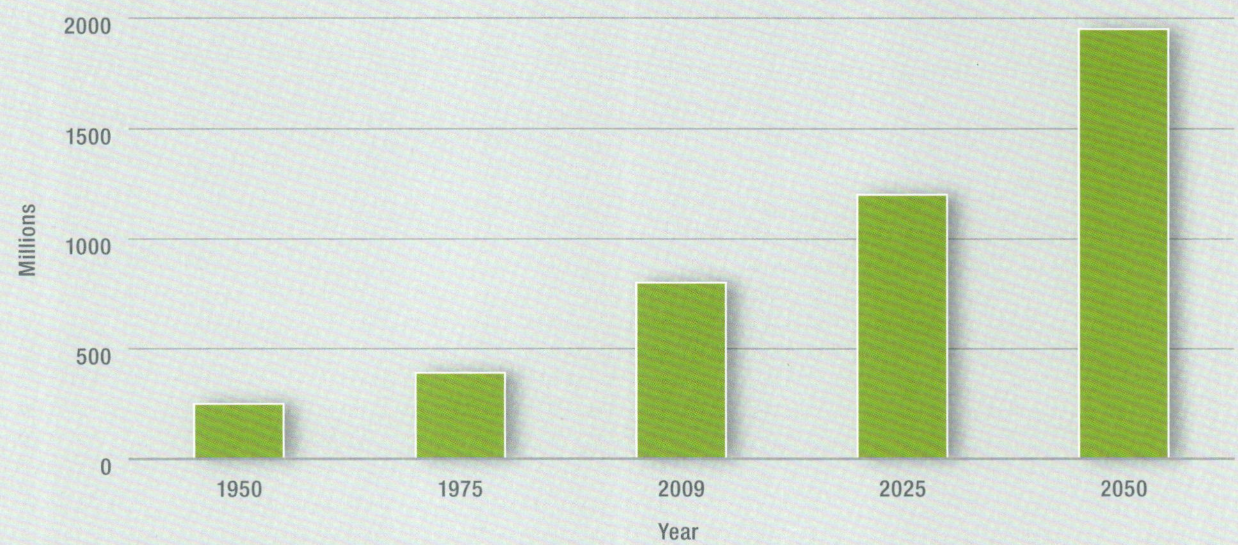


**FIG 1.1** World population aged 60 years or over, 1950–2050 *(5)*

In the majority of LMIC, and in some high-income countries, the growing prevalence and impact of dementia is not well understood. This is likely to be reflected in a lack of policy direction and programme development and in inappropriate allocation of funding. It is obvious that dementia, its consequences and responses can no longer be neglected and that it is time that dementia is considered part of the public health agenda by all stakeholders. Chronic diseases are gradually gaining attention in the public health arena. In September 2011, the United Nations convened a summit on non-communicable diseases at which it adopted a "political declaration" which included the acknowledgement that "the global burden and threat of non-communicable diseases constitutes one of the major challenges for development in the twenty-first century" (Item 1) and the recognition that "mental and neurological disorders, including Alzheimer's disease, are an important cause of morbidity and contribute to the global non-communicable disease burden" (Item 18) *(8)*.

# OBJECTIVES OF THE REPORT

The purpose of this report is to raise awareness of dementia as a public health priority, to articulate a public health approach, and to advocate for action at international and national levels based on the principles of inclusion, integration, equity and evidence.

The report provides information and aims to encourage country preparedness by strengthening or developing policy and implementing it through plans and programmes which enhance dementia care in order to improve the social well-being and quality of life of those living with dementia and their caregivers. It is hoped that this will lead to international and national advocacy efforts and the prioritization of dementia on the global health agenda. The target audiences are national and state ministries of health, policy-makers, and health and social sector planners, as well as academics and researchers. In addition, as a practical tool for improvement of dementia care and support, the report will be useful to organizations (both governmental and nongovernmental) involved in education and health and social service provision for older people and people with disabilities.

## DEVELOPMENT OF THE REPORT: METHODS

The information included in the report is derived from three primary sources:

- reports from four working groups (on epidemiology; national policies, plans and resources; awareness and the health workforce; and caregivers) that reviewed existing literature (including scientific literature and reports) and collected case examples relevant to each group;
- an online survey of available resources in 30 countries selected to represent high, middle and low incomes across the six WHO regions (Box 1.2); and
- additional information provided by stakeholders from 16 countries who attended a meeting in Geneva on 27–28 September 2011 (including representatives from public health, academia and advocacy groups).

## CONTENTS OF THE REPORT

The report has been developed to provide information to countries that will assist them to develop a response to dementia that is tailored to harmonize with their particular health and social care systems. The report is not comprehensive but is a selected review of information, evidence and current practices and policies. The management interventions (including psychosocial and pharmacological ones), have been covered in *WHO's mhGAP Intervention Guide for mental, neurological and substance use disorders for non-specialized health settings (9, 10)*.

The report provides an overview of the current impact of dementia worldwide. The main focus of the report is dementia in LMIC, where the impact of dementia is likely to be high and the current level of preparedness is particularly low. However, the problems described are by no means confined to developing countries and the report is useful for all countries. It reviews current resources and strategies in a number of countries and includes examples of national, regional and local interventions from which approaches can be drawn. Examples from specific countries used to illustrate various issues should not be viewed as assessments of countries overall health systems, nor should they be taken to mean that any country is more or less advanced in its approach to dementia than others.

Chapter 2 provides an overview of the global epidemiology of dementia. It provides a comprehensive evidence-based summary from epidemiological research pertaining to the global prevalence of dementia; the prevalence of young onset dementia; dementia subtypes; the global incidence of dementia; dementia-associated mortality; the global societal economic cost of dementia; and the etiology of dementia, and opportunities for prevention.

Chapter 3 includes a description of national-level approaches to dementia, including policy and plans where they exist, and key elements for developing a national approach. It reviews issues relating to the legal and financial support required for people with dementia and their caregivers, and highlights the ethical implications that affect all levels of decision-making and planning.

Chapter 4 examines the role of health and social support systems and their capacity to provide clinical management and long-term care. This chapter explores the issues around capacity-building of the health and social care workforce and how this can be enhanced.

Chapter 5 focuses on the caregivers of persons with dementia. It discusses the key issues that many caregivers experience as a result of providing long-term and, often, physically and psychologically demanding care. It identifies the barriers to accessing support, including the provision of care, and resources that could enable and improve effective informal care provision.

**Chapter 6** explores levels of awareness and understanding within the community and among health and social care providers. It identifies approaches to raising awareness and reducing stigma.

**Chapter 7** points the way forward. It discusses the need for action, the value of that action, and the themes or areas in which coordinated action is required.

In addition, a detailed appendix to this report is available on the Online appendix: http://www.who.int/mental_health/publications/dementia_report_2012.

Overall, this report provides the foundation for identifying dementia as a public health priority and calls for action. It provides the knowledge base for global and national responses, and aims to support governments, policy-makers and other stakeholders in addressing the impact of the growing threat to global health due to dementia. It identifies approaches and opportunities that can make health and social care systems dementia-informed and responsive. All these actions are feasible in some manner, especially in many LMIC. Appropriate and effective efforts put in place today will pay off for the coming generations.

**BOX 1.2**

## WHO DEMENTIA SURVEY METHODOLOGY

Aim: To gather information on current resources, gaps and initiatives for supporting dementia in a range of countries representing high, middle and low income levels.

Methods:

- The survey targeted 41 countries representing high, middle and low incomes and large and smaller populations in the six WHO regions, and received 30 (73%) responses.
- It was piloted in Australia and the Dominican Republic.
- Respondents were key personnel in Alzheimer organizations in 28 countries (in consultation with expert informants as necessary). Two respondents from countries without an Alzheimer organization were senior health professionals.
- The domains covered were awareness, understanding and attitudes; policies; programmes; financial support; legislation; primary and specialist health care; long-term care (community, residential, palliative); workforce education; caregiver support; and the role of civil society organizations.
- Limitations of the survey were that countries were selected from among membership of Alzheimer's Disease International, and that information provided by country representatives consisted of best estimates.

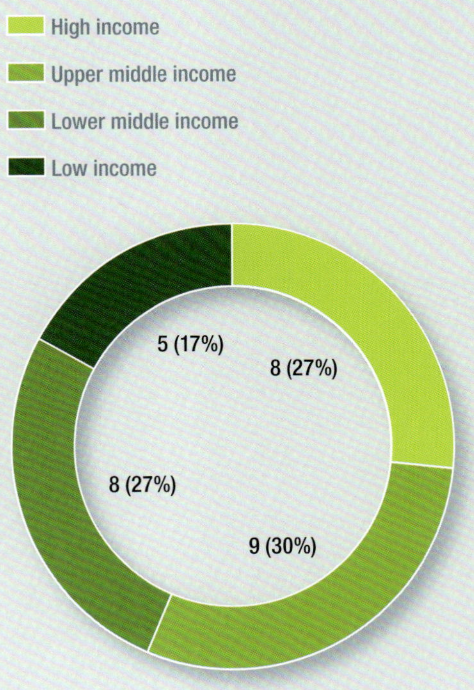


Title: Number (%) of responding countries by World Bank Income Group

CHAPTER 2

# EPIDEMIOLOGY OF DEMENTIA

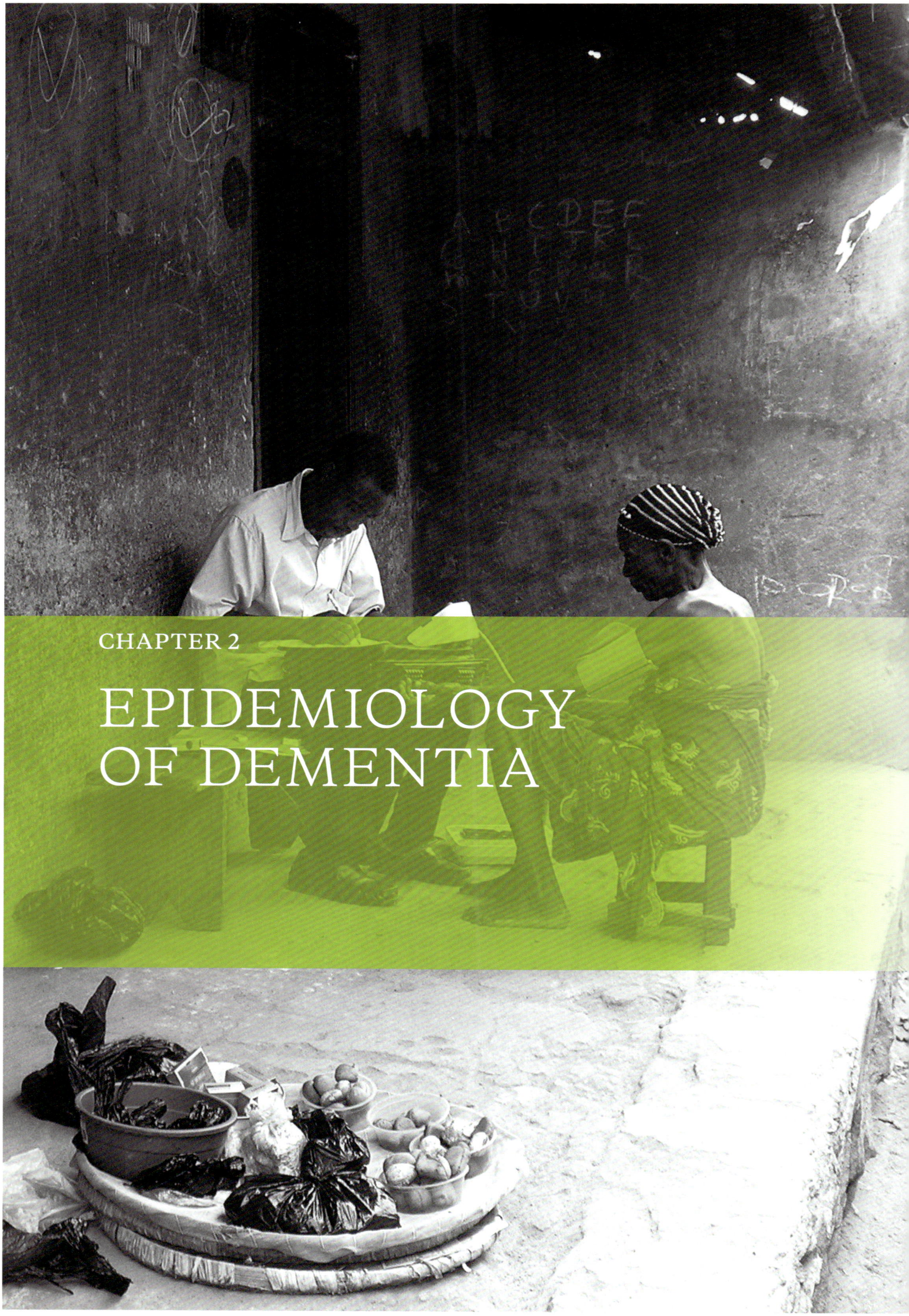

Dementia mainly affects older people, although there is growing awareness of cases that start before the age of 65. Population ageing is having a profound impact on the emergence of the global dementia epidemic, influencing awareness and driving demand for services. Particularly rapid increases in the numbers and proportions of older people are forecast for China, India and Latin America *(11)*. By 2050 people aged 60 and over will account for 22% of the world's population, four-fifths living in Africa, Asia or Latin America. As yet, public and policy-maker awareness of dementia and health system preparedness for it are much more limited in these regions where the epidemic will be concentrated in the coming decades. It is therefore important to track the global prevalence and impact of this burdensome condition and its regional distribution in the context of rapidly unfolding demographic and health transitions.

## GLOBAL PREVALENCE OF DEMENTIA

### LATE ONSET DEMENTIA

In 2005, Alzheimer's Disease International (ADI) commissioned a panel of experts to review all available epidemiological data and reach a consensus estimate of prevalence in each of 14 world regions *(12)*. The panel estimated 24.3 million people aged 60 years and over with dementia in 2001, 60% living in LMIC. Each year, 4.6 million new cases were predicted, with numbers affected nearly doubling every 20 years to reach 81.1 million by 2040. Incidence was estimated from prevalence and mortality. The estimates were provisional, due to limited data *(12)*. Coverage was good in Europe, North America, and in developed Asia-Pacific countries. Studies from China and India were too few and estimates too variable to provide a consistent overview. There was a dearth of studies from Latin America *(13–15)*, Africa *(16)*, Eastern Europe, Russia and the Middle East, and a consequent reliance on the consensus judgement of the international expert panel. This supported a tendency, noted in the few LMIC studies available at that time, for the age-specific prevalence of dementia to be lower in developing countries than in developed ones *(16–18)*.

Global prevalence is being reappraised for the revision of the *Global burden of disease* (GBD) study 2010 (http: //www.globalburden.org/), with findings summarized in ADI's 2009 *World Alzheimer Report (3)*. The evidence base was expanded considerably with more studies from LMIC and from other regions and groups previously underrepresented in the literature. Enhancements included a fully systematic review of the world literature on the prevalence of dementia (1980–2009) in 21 GBD regions, a critical appraisal of study quality, and an attempt, where possible, to generate regional estimates from quantitative meta-analysis. Details of the methodology can be found in the web appendix[1].

#### SEARCH RESULTS

The search yielded abstracts for 2017 publications. Of these, 155 publications (describing 167 studies) were considered to be provisionally eligible. For 20 of these publications, it was not possible to confirm eligibility. A full list of included and excluded publications is provided in the web appendix[1]. Finally, 135 publications (describing 147 studies) were fully eligible for inclusion in the review.

#### COVERAGE

Good-to-reasonable coverage was identified for 11 of the 21 GBD regions (Tables 2.1 and 2.2). Western Europe (56 studies) and East Asia (34 studies) accounted for most of the world's studies. The next best represented region was Asia Pacific High Income (22 studies), followed by North America (13 studies), and Latin America (11 studies – comprising three in the Andean, four in the Central, one in the Southern and three in the Tropical Latin America region). Other regions with reasonable coverage were South Asia (7 studies), South-East Asia (5 studies) and Australasia (4 studies). Five regions were sparsely covered; the Caribbean (4 studies as three of the four studies were conducted in Cuba, and the other in the Dominican Republic, thus only two countries were covered from the region), Central Europe (4 studies), North Africa / Middle East (2 studies), Eastern Europe (1 study) and Western sub-Saharan Africa (2 studies) and Southern sub-Saharan Africa (1 study). No eligible studies were identified for Central and Eastern sub-Saharan Africa, or for Central Asia. Figure 2.1, summarizing the annual number of prevalence studies according to the median year in which data were collected, indicates a large and sustained increase in studies conducted in LMIC since the mid-1990s, while studies in high-income countries peaked in the early 1990s and declined sharply thereafter; 27% of studies in high-income countries (chiefly in Europe and North America) were conducted in the 1980s, 63% in the 1990s and 10% in the 2000s.

1. http://www.who.int/mental_health/publications/dementia_report_2012

## THE QUALITY OF INCLUDED STUDIES

The quality of the studies included in the survey was evaluated on the basis of combined index, study design, scope of diagnostic assessment, sample size, response proportion and overall quality. Details can be found online in the web appendix to this report[1].

## META-ANALYSIS OF DEMENTIA PREVALENCE WITHIN GBD REGIONS

There were sufficient studies of good quality to conduct meta-analyses for 11 of the 21 GBD regions; Western Europe, North America, Latin America (combining Andean, Central, Southern and Tropical regions), Asia Pacific high-income, Australasia, East Asia, South-East Asia and South Asia. For Latin America, we considered it pragmatic and appropriate to pool studies from across the four GBD regions to conduct a single continent-wide meta-analysis. Given that the North American region comprised just Canada and the USA, and that Canada was represented by a large and well-conducted survey on a nationally representative sample *(19)*, the national prevalence figures for Canada were applied to Canada and the USA studies were meta-analysed to generate estimates for that country.

## MODELLING THE PREVALENCE OF DEMENTIA

Age-specific and age- and sex-specific meta-analysed dementia prevalence estimates are described for each region in Table 2.1. Prevalence increased exponentially with age in each region, doubling with every 5.5 year increment in age in Asia Pacific, Latin America and North America, with every 5.6 year increment in East Asia, every 6.3 years in South Asia and Western Europe, and every 6.7 years in Australasia and South-East Asia. In all regions other than Asia Pacific and North America, the predicted prevalence for men was lower (by 19–29%) than that for women. There was a tendency in all regions for the divergence in prevalence between men and women to increase with increasing age; however, this was statistically significant only for the Asia Pacific region. There was statistically significant heterogeneity (variation in prevalence between studies within regions) for all regions other than South-East.

## GENERATION OF PREVALENCE ESTIMATES FOR OTHER GBD REGIONS

Where it was impractical to conduct a meta-analysis due to insufficient data, the default option was to apply relevant estimates from the Delphi consensus of 2005, representing the best available estimates of likely dementia prevalence in those regions *(12)*. For a full description of the strategies used, see online appendix[1].

## ESTIMATED PREVALENCE OF DEMENTIA

Estimated prevalence of dementia for all those aged 60 years and over, age-standardized to the Western Europe population structure, can be compared directly between the 21 GBD regions (Tables 2.1 and 2.2 and Figure 2.2). There is a four-fold variation, from 2.07% (West sub-Saharan Africa) to 8.50% (Latin America). However, most of the estimated age-standardized prevalence figures lie in a band between 5% and 7%. The major source of variation is the very low estimated prevalence for the four regions of sub-Saharan Africa.

## ESTIMATION OF NUMBERS OF PEOPLE WITH DEMENTIA

Having applied the age-specific, or age- and sex-specific, prevalence estimates to UN population projections, it was estimated that 35.6 million people worldwide were living with dementia in 2010 (Table 2.3). Western Europe is the GBD region with the highest number of people with dementia (7.0 million), closely followed by East Asia with 5.5 million, South Asia with 4.5 million and North America with 4.4 million. The nine countries with the largest number of people with dementia in 2010 (1 million or more) were China (5.4 million), USA (3.9 million), India (3.7 million), Japan (2.5 million), Germany (1.5 million), Russia (1.2 million), France (1.1 million), Italy (1.1 million) and Brazil (1.0 million).

The total number of people with dementia is projected to almost double every 20 years, to 65.7 million in 2030 and 115.4 million in 2050. Much of the increase is attributable to increases in the numbers of people with dementia in LMIC (Figure 2.3); in 2010, 57.7% of all people with dementia lived in LMIC, and this proportion is expected to rise to 63.4% in 2030 and 70.5% in 2050. The projections are driven mainly by population growth and demographic ageing (Table 2.3). World regions fall into three broad groups. High-income countries start from a high base, but will experience only a moderate proportionate increase – a 40% increase in Europe, 63% in North America, 77% in the southern Latin American cone and 89% in the developed Asia Pacific countries. Other parts of Latin America and North Africa and the Middle East start from a low base but will experience a particularly rapid increase – 134–146% in the rest of Latin America, and 125% in North Africa and the Middle East. China, India and their neighbours in South Asia and Western Pacific start from a high base and will also experience rapid growth – 107% in South Asia and 117% in East Asia. Projected increases for sub-Saharan Africa (70–94%) are modest and are consistent with limited demographic ageing in view of persistently high child mortality and the effects of the HIV epidemic.

1. http://www.who.int/mental_health/publications/dementia_report_2012

| GBD region | Number of studies | | Sex | Age group (years) | | | | | | | Standardised prevalence[1], for those aged 60 and over |
|---|---|---|---|---|---|---|---|---|---|---|---|
| | Potentially eligible studies | Used in meta-analysis (age-specific, age- and sex specific) | | 60–64 | 65–69 | 70–74 | 75–79 | 80–84 | 85–89 | 90+ | |
| **ASIA** | | | | | | | | | | | |
| Australasia | 4 | 3, 0 | All | 1.8 | 2.8 | 4.5 | 7.5 | 12.5 | 20.3 | 38.3 | 6.91* |
| Asia Pacific, High Income | 22 | 14, 10 | M | 1.4 | 2.3 | 3.8 | 6.4 | 10.9 | 18 | 34.9 | 6.30* |
| | | | F | 0.9 | 1.7 | 3.1 | 6.0 | 11.7 | 21.7 | 49.2 | |
| | | | All | 1.0 | 1.7 | 2.9 | 5.5 | 10.3 | 18.5 | 40.1 | 5.57 |
| Asia, East | 34 | 34, 31 | M | 0.8 | 1.3 | 2.2 | 4.0 | 7.3 | 16.7 | 26.4 | 4.98* |
| | | | F | 0.9 | 1.6 | 2.9 | 5.3 | 10.0 | 17.9 | 38.7 | |
| | | | All | 0.7 | 1.2 | 3.1 | 4.0 | 7.4 | 13.3 | 28.7 | 4.19 |
| Asia, South | 8 | 7, 6 | M | 1.0 | 1.7 | 2.9 | 5.3 | 9.4 | 16.4 | 33.7 | 5.65* |
| | | | F | 1.5 | 2.3 | 3.8 | 6.5 | 11 | 18.1 | 35.1 | |
| | | | All | 1.3 | 2.1 | 3.5 | 6.1 | 10.6 | 17.8 | 35.4 | 5.78 |
| Asia, Southeast | 6 | 5, 2 | M | 1.7 | 2.6 | 4.0 | 6.2 | 9.8 | 15 | 26.4 | 7.63 |
| | | | F | 1.8 | 3.0 | 5.1 | 9.0 | 15.9 | 27.2 | 54.9 | |
| | | | All | 1.6 | 2.6 | 4.2 | 6.9 | 11.6 | 18.7 | 35.4 | 6.38* |
| **EUROPE** | | | | | | | | | | | |
| Europe, Western | 56 | 52, 46 | M | 1.4 | 2.3 | 3.7 | 6.3 | 10.6 | 17.4 | 33.4 | 7.29* |
| | | | F | 1.9 | 3.0 | 5.0 | 8.6 | 14.8 | 24.7 | 48.3 | |
| | | | All | 1.6 | 2.6 | 4.3 | 7.4 | 12.9 | 21.7 | 43.1 | 6.92 |
| **THE AMERICAS** | | | | | | | | | | | |
| North America (USA only) | 11 | 8, 6 | M | 1.3 | 2.1 | 3.7 | 6.8 | 12.3 | 21.6 | 45.2 | 6.77* |
| | | | F | 1.0 | 1.8 | 3.3 | 6.4 | 12.5 | 23.2 | 52.7 | |
| | | | All | 1.1 | 1.9 | 3.4 | 6.3 | 11.9 | 21.7 | 47.5 | 6.46 |
| Latin America | 11 | 11, 10 | M | 1.0 | 1.9 | 3.7 | 7.0 | 13.0 | 24.3 | 55.0 | 8.50* |
| | | | F | 1.0 | 2.0 | 4.2 | 8.4 | 16.4 | 32.5 | 79.5 | |
| | | | All | 1.3 | 2.4 | 4.5 | 8.4 | 15.4 | 28.6 | 63.9 | 8.48 |

1. Standardized for age, or for age and sex (*)

TABLE 2.1 Meta-analysed estimates of dementia prevalence (%), generated from Poisson random effects models, by Global Burden of Disease region

| GBD region | Sources of prevalence data used to calculate regional weighted average | Age group (years) | | | | | | Age-standardised prevalence for all those aged 60 years and over |
|---|---|---|---|---|---|---|---|---|
| | | 60–64 | 65–69 | 70–74 | 75–79 | 80–84 | 85+ | |
| **ASIA** | | | | | | | | |
| Asia, Central | EUR B, EUR C | 0.9 | 1.3 | 3.2 | 5.8 | 12.1 | 24.7 | 5.75 |
| Oceania | WPR B | 0.6 | 1.8 | 3.7 | 7.0 | 14.4 | 26.2 | 6.46 |
| **EUROPE** | | | | | | | | |
| Europe, Central | EUR A, EUR B | 0.9 | 1.3 | 3.3 | 5.8 | 12.2 | 24.7 | 5.78 |
| Europe, Eastern | EUR C | 0.9 | 1.3 | 3.2 | 5.8 | 11.8 | 24.5 | 5.70 |
| **THE AMERICAS** | | | | | | | | |
| Caribbean | AMR B, AMR D, Cuba *(20, 21)*, Dominican Republic *(20)* | 1.3 | 2.6 | 4.9 | 8.5 | 16.0 | 33.2 | 8.12 |
| **AFRICA** | | | | | | | | |
| North Africa/ Middle East | EMR B, AFR D, Egypt *(22)* | 1.0 | 1.6 | 3.5 | 6.0 | 12.9 | 23.0 | 5.85 |
| Sub-Saharan Africa, Central | AFR D, AFR E | 0.5 | 0.9 | 1.8 | 3.5 | 6.4 | 13.8 | 3.25 |
| Sub-Saharan Africa, East | AFR E, AFR D, EMR D | 0.6 | 1.2 | 2.3 | 4.3 | 8.2 | 16.3 | 4.00 |
| Sub-Saharan Africa, Southern | | 0.5 | 1.0 | 1.9 | 3.8 | 7.0 | 14.9 | 3.51 |
| Sub-Saharan Africa, West | Nigeria *(16)* | 0.3 | 0.86 | | 2.72 | | 9.59 | 2.07 |

Note: AFR D, WHO African Region with high child and high adult mortality; AFR E, WHO African Region with high child and very high adult mortality; AMR B, WHO Region of the Americas with low child and low adult mortality; AMR D, WHO Region of the Americas with high child and high adult mortality; EMR B, WHO Eastern Mediterranean Region with low child and low adult mortality; EMR D, WHO Eastern Mediterranean Region with high child and high adult mortality; EUR A, WHO European Region with very low child and very low adult mortality; EUR B, WHO European Region with low child and low adult mortality; EUR C, WHO European Region with low child and high adult mortality; WPR B, WHO Western Pacific Region with low child and low adult mortality.

TABLE 2.2 Estimates of dementia prevalence (%) for Global Burden of Disease regions where it was not possible to carry out a quantitative meta-analysis

## YOUNG ONSET DEMENTIA

Young onset dementia (YOD), defined typically as onset before the age of 65 years, is a rare condition. Few population-based surveys have been carried out, since large sample sizes are needed to estimate prevalence with precision. Instead, researchers typically conduct registry-based studies, reporting prevalence calculated as the number of cases known to local service providers divided by the total local population from the census. The assumption is that all of those with YOD seek help early in the disease course. This is not always the case, and therefore such studies will underestimate the true prevalence of dementia.

### REVIEW

The European Collaboration on Dementia group (EuroCoDe) carried out a systematic review of prevalence of YOD *(23)*. In addition to two registry-based studies from the United Kingdom, the group identified a registry-based study from the USA *(24)*, and a population-based survey of late-onset dementia from Rotterdam, Netherlands, in which the youngest age group was 55–59 years *(25)*. The reviewers commented on the scarcity of data and variability of estimates, and did not attempt a meta-analysis. A Delphi consensus had previously been attempted for the *Dementia UK* report *(26)*, using the two United Kingdom studies, one carried out in Cambridgeshire *(27)*, and the other in four London boroughs *(28)*. The prevalence of persons aged 45–64 was, for males, 120 / 100000 in London and 101 / 100000 in Cambridgeshire; and for females 77 / 100000 in London and 61 / 100000 in Cambridgeshire. For YOD, as with late onset dementia, the expert consensus was that prevalence increased exponentially with increasing age, roughly doubling every five years from 9 / 100000 at age 30 to 156 / 100000 at age 60–64

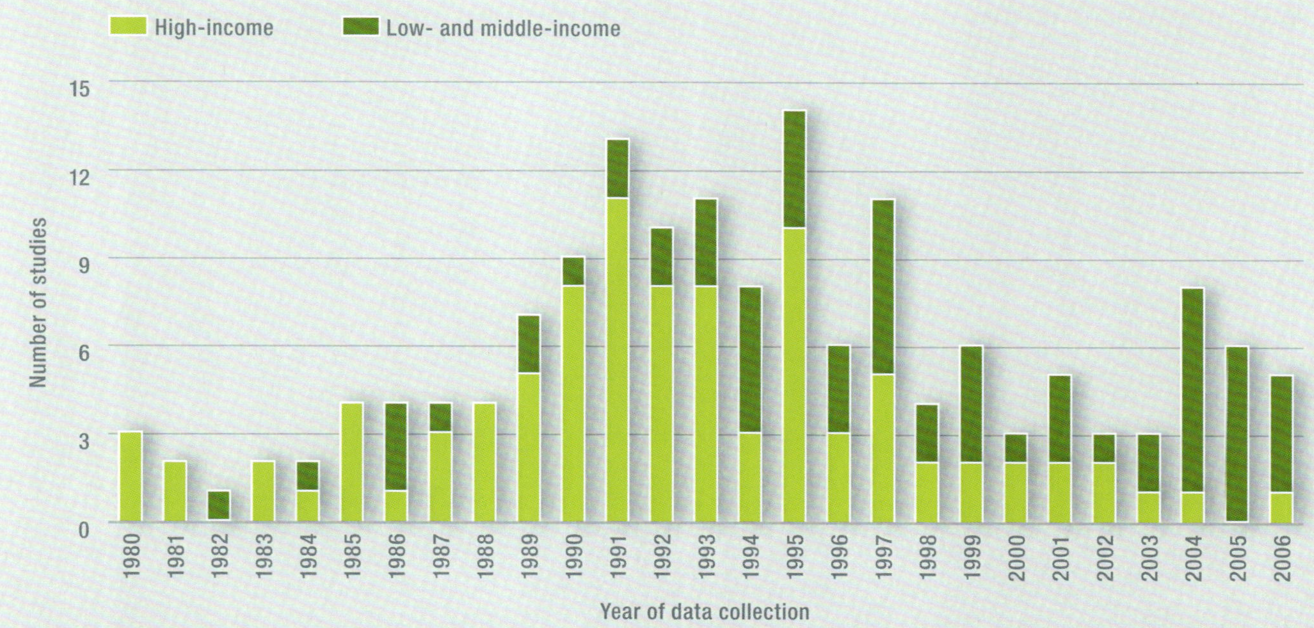


FIG 2.1 Number of prevalence studies, by year of data collection and income level of the country where the research was carried out

years. Two-thirds (68%) of all young onset cases were aged 55 and over. Among this larger, middle-aged group of people with YOD, males predominated over females with a gender ratio of 1.7 to 1.

The consensus group's estimate for 60–64 years (156 / 100 000, or 0.16%) is one-ninth rather than, as expected, one half of the late-onset prevalence for the next five-year age band (1.3% for those aged 65–69). This discrepancy is likely to be artefactual, arising from an underestimation of population prevalence in the YOD studies, which ascertained cases from service contact only. This explanation is supported by the Rotterdam population-based survey prevalence of 423 / 100 000 for those aged 55–59 and 418 / 100 000 for those aged 60–64 *(25)*. Thus, there may be an underestimation by registry-based studies of the true prevalence of YOD by a factor of 2.5 to fourfold. While it was estimated that YOD accounts for only 2.2% of all people with dementia in the United Kingdom *(26)*, the true proportion may be closer to 6–9%.

It is sometimes suggested, chiefly on the grounds of lower life expectancies at birth, that ageing begins earlier in LMIC. These differences are mainly accounted for by early life mortality and there is little evidence that YOD is more common in LMIC. Three prevalence studies from India included participants aged less than 65 years, and prevalences of YOD were as low as those seen in high-income population-based surveys: 328 / 100 000 (60–64 years) in Kerala *(24)*, 249 / 100 000 in Ballabgarh (55–64 years) *(18)*, and 63 / 100 000 (50–59 years) and 280 / 100 000 (60–64 years) in Mumbai *(30)*. However, this statement must be qualified given the likely impact of the HIV epidemic which is concentrated among younger people in low-income countries, particularly in southern and eastern Africa. HIV-associated dementia is an AIDS-defining illness, with a prevalence of 15–30% in untreated populations, presenting with neurocognitive impairments (forgetfulness, poor concentration and slowed mental processing), emotional disturbances (agitation, apathy), and motor dysfunction. The condition is also seen among those receiving Highly Active Antiretroviral Therapy (HAART) with a prevalence of 10% and an annual incidence of 1% *(31, 32)*. Beyond HIV-associated dementia, HIV-associated neurocognitive disorder (HAND) has a prevalence of 20–30%. Higher prevalences have been seen among people accessing HIV care in high HIV seroprevalence sub-Saharan African countries (e.g. 42% with HAND and 25% with HIV-associated dementia in those starting HAART in primary care centres in Cape Town, South Africa) *(33)*. Cognitive disorder in HIV is particularly important in view of associations with poor adherence to HAART, faster disease progression, and mortality *(34)*. It is difficult to quantify the impact on numbers of people with dementia and on the age distribution of dementia cases in the region. However, given an HIV adult seroprevalence of 15–25% in southern African countries, this will be considerable, and it is conceivable that most dementia cases may be younger people with HIV-associated dementia.

## DISCUSSION - PREVALENCE OF DEMENTIA

The current estimates provide an indication of the numbers of people aged 60 years and over with dementia worldwide and in different world regions. There is much more uncertainty as to the prevalence of YOD but, if such cases were to be included, the total numbers affected might be up to 6–9% higher. The current estimates for the prevalence of dementia among those aged 60 years and over are approximately 10% higher than those from the earlier

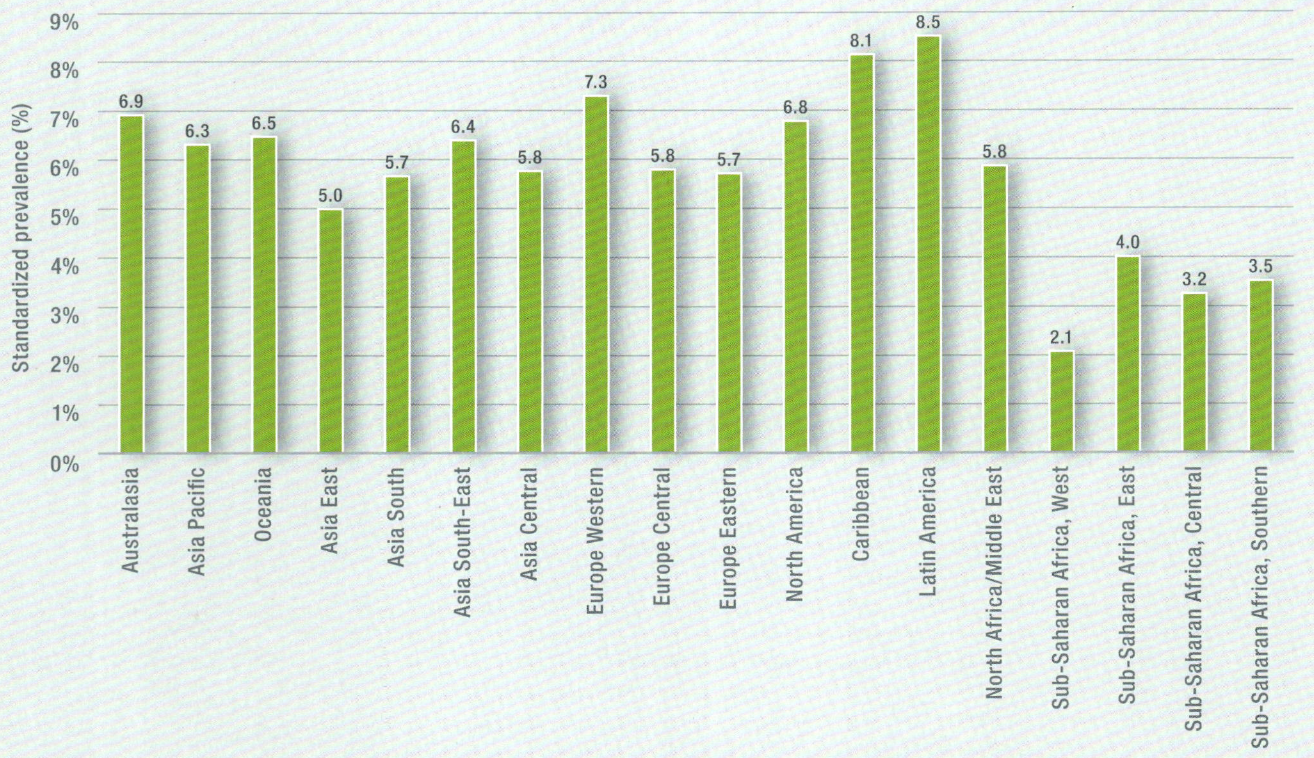


FIG 2.2 Estimated prevalence of dementia for persons aged 60 and over, standardized to Western Europe population, by Global Burden of Disease region

ADI Delphi consensus *(11)*, accounted for by a higher age-standardized prevalence for South Asia (5.7% versus 3.4%), Western Europe (7.3% versus 5.9%) and the Latin American regions (8.5% versus 7.3%). These increases were partly offset by the lower estimated prevalence for East Asia (5.0% versus 6.5%). The new estimates are likely to be an improvement on those provided earlier, given the extension in the evidence base from LMIC. It was possible to include seven studies from South Asia, 52 from Western Europe, 34 from East Asia and 11 from Latin America in the regional meta-analyses. There was previously just one prevalence study available from Latin America *(13)*. The evidence base from China was considerably extended by a recent systematic review that included data from publications previously available only in Chinese journals *(35)*. The previous estimates for South Asia were perhaps disproportionately influenced by one large study, from rural Ballabgarh in northern India, which recorded an unusually low prevalence *(18)*. Earlier estimates for Europe *(12)* were strongly influenced by two previous reviews by the European Community Concerted Action on the Epidemiology and Prevention of Dementia Group (EURODEM) *(36, 37)*. The current systematic review is much more comprehensive, and the new estimates coincide with the 7.1% prevalence derived from a recent systematic review by the EuroCoDe group *(23)*.

Data was insufficient for certain regions, particularly Eastern Europe, North Africa, the Middle East, Russia, and sub-Saharan Africa (see also the section on Coverage). As such, the estimates must still be considered provisional. The current estimates have drawn on previous Delphi consensus estimates for these regions. A limitation of this review could be using two methodologies to quantify prevalence estimates for different GBD regions, i.e. meta-analysis for 11 out of 21 regions where sufficient studies were available and for others (due to insufficient data), use of relevant estimates from the Delphi consensus. Meta-analysis methods that allow estimates for regions without data by borrowing strength from those with data would allow updated estimates for all regions. This also emphasizes the need of more data of good quality for the GBD regions where sufficient studies were not available.

The low prevalences for sub-Saharan Africa are mainly determined by the one good-quality study (Ibadan, Nigeria) that was available when the review was conducted in 2009 *(16)*. Subsequent studies from francophone countries in western and central Africa *(38–40)*, and one further study from northern Nigeria *(41)* suggest a more variable prevalence, higher in urban than in rural sites, and higher in central compared with western Africa. The Nigerian study recorded a low prevalence that is consistent with findings from the earlier USA/Nigeria study (2.4% for those aged 65 and over, age-stan-

| GBD region | Population over 60 years (millions, 2010) | Crude estimated prevalence (%, 2010) | Number of people with dementia (millions) | | | Proportionate increases (%) | |
|---|---|---|---|---|---|---|---|
| | | | 2010 | 2030 | 2050 | 2010–2030 | 2010–2050 |
| **ASIA** | **406.55** | **3.9** | **15.94** | **33.04** | **60.92** | **107** | **282** |
| Australasia | 4.82 | 6.4 | 0.31 | 0.53 | 0.79 | 71 | 157 |
| Asia Pacific | 46.63 | 6.1 | 2.83 | 5.36 | 7.03 | 89 | 148 |
| Oceania | 0.49 | 4.0 | 0.02 | 0.04 | 0.10 | 100 | 400 |
| Asia, Central | 7.16 | 4.6 | 0.33 | 0.56 | 1.19 | 70 | 261 |
| Asia, East | 171.61 | 3.2 | 5.49 | 11.93 | 22.54 | 117 | 311 |
| Asia, South | 124.61 | 3.6 | 4.48 | 9.31 | 18.12 | 108 | 304 |
| Asia, Southeast | 51.22 | 4.8 | 2.48 | 5.30 | 11.13 | 114 | 349 |
| **EUROPE** | **160.18** | **6.2** | **9.95** | **13.95** | **18.65** | **40** | **87** |
| Europe, Western | 97.27 | 7.2 | 6.98 | 10.03 | 13.44 | 44 | 93 |
| Europe, Central | 23.61 | 4.7 | 1.10 | 1.57 | 2.10 | 43 | 91 |
| Europe, East | 39.30 | 4.8 | 1.87 | 2.36 | 3.10 | 26 | 66 |
| **THE AMERICAS** | **120.74** | **6.5** | **7.82** | **14.78** | **27.08** | **89** | **246** |
| North America | 63.67 | 6.9 | 4.38 | 7.13 | 11.01 | 63 | 151 |
| Caribbean | 5.06 | 6.5 | 0.33 | 0.62 | 1.04 | 88 | 215 |
| Latin America, Andean | 4.51 | 5.6 | 0.25 | 0.59 | 1.29 | 136 | 416 |
| Latin America, Central | 19.54 | 6.1 | 1.19 | 2.79 | 6.37 | 134 | 435 |
| Latin America, Southern | 8.74 | 7.0 | 0.61 | 1.08 | 1.83 | 77 | 200 |
| Latin America, Tropical | 19.23 | 5.5 | 1.05 | 2.58 | 5.54 | 146 | 428 |
| **AFRICA** | **71.07** | **2.6** | **1.86** | **3.92** | **8.74** | **111** | **370** |
| North Africa/ Middle East | 31.11 | 3.7 | 1.15 | 2.59 | 6.19 | 125 | 438 |
| Sub-Saharan Africa, Central | 3.93 | 1.8 | 0.07 | 0.12 | 0.24 | 71 | 243 |
| Sub-Saharan Africa, East | 16.03 | 2.3 | 0.36 | 0.69 | 1.38 | 92 | 283 |
| Sub-Saharan Africa, Southern | 4.66 | 2.1 | 0.10 | 0.17 | 0.20 | 70 | 100 |
| Sub-Saharan Africa, West | 15.33 | 1.2 | 0.18 | 0.35 | 0.72 | 94 | 300 |
| **WORLD** | **758.54** | **4.7** | **35.56** | **65.69** | **115.38** | **85** | **225** |

TABLE 2.3 Total population over 60, crude estimated prevalence of dementia (2010), estimated number of people with dementia (2010, 2030 and 2050) and proportionate increases (2010–2030 and 2010–2050) by Global Burden of Disease region

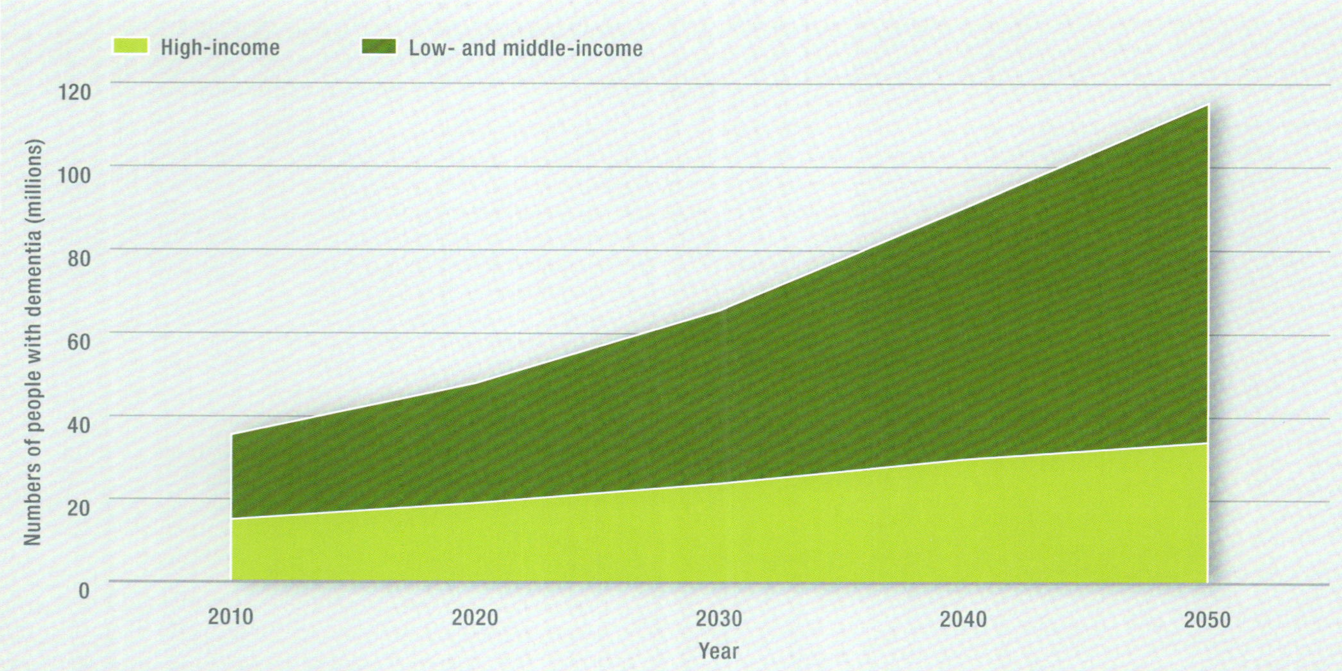


FIG 2.3 Growth in numbers of people with dementia in high-income and low- and middle-income countries

dardized to Western Europe, with an age-standardized prevalence of 1.9% for those aged 60 and over assuming that the prevalence for those aged 60–64, which was not assessed, was half that of those aged 65–74) *(41)*. Prevalence was similarly low in rural Benin (2.4% age-standardized for age 65+ and 2.0% for age 60+ similarly estimated) *(38)*. The prevalence in urban Benin was higher (4.3% and 3.5%) *(40)* and that recorded in cities in the Central African Republic (10.1% and 8.2%) and the Republic of the Congo (7.2% and 6.0%) was substantially higher *(39)*.

Current evidence therefore challenges the previous consensus that the prevalence of dementia was lower in LMIC *(17)*, and strikingly so in some studies *(16, 18)*. Methodological factors may be implicated. In the 10/66 Dementia Research Group studies (Box 2.1), the group's 10/66 dementia diagnosis – developed, calibrated and validated in a 26-site pilot study *(42)* – was both more prevalent than that according to DSM-IV criteria, and more consistent between sites. The prevalence of DSM-IV dementia was particularly low in rural and less developed sites *(20)*. It may be that milder dementia is under-detected in LMIC because of low awareness, high levels of support routinely provided to older people, and reluctance to report failings to outsiders, which could all contribute to difficulties in establishing the DSM-IV criterion of social and occupational impairment *(18, 20)*. In Cuba, the criterion validity of the 10/66 diagnosis was superior to that of DSM-IV which selectively missed mild and moderate cases *(43)*. In India, the predictive validity of the 10/66 diagnosis was supported by high mortality after three years of follow-up, with survivors showing expected progression of cognitive impairment, disability and needs for care *(44)*; this suggested that the true prevalence at baseline was likely to be much closer to the 7.5% recorded for 10/66 dementia than the 0.9% prevalence according to DSM-IV criteria *(20)*.

## DEMENTIA SUBTYPES

The four commonest subtypes in order of frequency are Alzheimer's disease, vascular dementia (VaD), dementia with Lewy bodies (DLB), and frontotemporal dementia (FTD). Estimates of the proportion of dementia cases attributable to each of these must be interpreted with caution since these are clinical diagnoses based on typical patterns of onset and course. It is difficult, particularly in epidemiological studies, to gather all the necessary information for accurate subtype diagnosis. Neuroimaging biomarkers are routinely available for cerebrovascular disease, but imaging of amyloid plaques has only recently become available as a research technique. Evidence from neuropathological studies challenges the notion of discrete subtypes. Mixed pathologies are much more common than "pure" ones – particularly for Alzheimer's disease and VaD, and Alzheimer's disease and DLB *(45)*. In one case series of over 1 000 post mortems, while 86% of all those with dementia had pathology related to Alzheimer's disease, only 43% had pure Alzheimer's disease, 26% had mixed Alzheimer's disease and cerebrovascular pathology, and 10% had Alzheimer's disease with cortical Lewy bodies *(46)*. Findings were similar for those who had been given a clinical diagnosis of Alzheimer's disease: "pure" VaD was comparatively rare (7.3%), and uncommon subtypes of dementia, including FTD, tended to be misdiagnosed in life as Alzheimer's disease *(46)*. Furthermore, the relationship between Alzheimer's disease neuropathology and dementia syndrome is less clear-cut than previously thought. Some individuals with advanced pathology do not develop dementia, and cerebrovascular disease may be an important co-factor determining dementia onset *(45, 47)*. Therefore, estimates of the proportion of cases accounted for by Alzheimer's disease, VaD, mixed dementia, DLB, FTD and other dementias represent, at best, the relative prominence of these different pathologies.

## REVIEW

The most sophisticated analysis of dementia subtype was that carried out for the *Dementia UK* report. Authors estimated the proportion of dementia cases accounted for by different subtypes according to age and sex, using a Delphi consensus of United Kingdom and other European evidence *(26)*. Three of six United Kingdom population-based studies of late-onset dementia included information on subtype diagnoses (Alzheimer's disease, VaD or mixed dementia and "other") *(48–50)*. A more recent community-based study *(51)* provided information on the relative frequency of a wider range of subtypes; Alzheimer's disease (41%), VaD (32%), dementia in Parkinson's Disease (3%), FTD (3%) and DLB (8%); Only the EURODEM meta-analysis of studies in the 1990s provided gender- as well as age-specific proportions with Alzheimer's disease and VaD *(37)*. In that study, while the proportion with Alzheimer's disease among females remained constant at around 70%, among men the proportion increased progressively from 38% among those aged 65–69 years to 80% in those over 90 years of age. Two YOD studies included detailed information on the full range of dementia subtypes, based on specialist dementia clinic assessments *(27, 28)*. Two further YOD studies provided limited information on the relative frequency of Alzheimer's disease, VaD and mixed dementia *(52, 53)*.

The results indicate that the FTD is a common subtype in YOD, particularly among men among whom it is the commonest subtype up to age 55 (Figures 2.4a and 2.4b). Vascular dementia is also relatively more common among men aged 45–75 years of age. While the proportion of dementia cases attributable to Alzheimer's disease, the commonest subtype overall, is relatively constant among women varying between 40–60% across the age range from 30 years and over, among men the proportion increases steadily with age from around 20% at age 30 to around 70% at ages 95 and over.

Studies in developed countries have consistently reported Alzheimer's disease to be more prevalent than VaD. Early surveys from South-East Asia were an exception, though more recent studies suggest that the pattern may now have reversed *(54)*. This may be due to increasing longevity and better physical health. Alzheimer's disease, with typically a later age of onset than VaD, increases as the number of very old people increases. Better physical health reduces cerebrovascular disease and hence the numbers with VaD. These changes also tend to shift the sex ratio towards a preponderance of female cases.

**BOX 2.1**

### THE 10/66 DEMENTIA RESEARCH GROUP'S POPULATION-BASED STUDIES

Alzheimer's Disease International's 10/66 Dementia Research Group has conducted population-based surveys (2003–2007) of dementia prevalence and impact in 14 catchment areas in 10 LMIC (Brazil, China, Cuba, Dominican Republic, India, Mexico, Nigeria, Peru, Puerto Rico and Venezuela). Cross-sectional, comprehensive, one-phase surveys were conducted of all residents aged 65 years and over of geographically defined catchment areas in each centre with a sample size of between 1 000 and 3 000 (generally 2 000) in each of the countries. Each study uses the same core minimum data set with cross-culturally validated assessments (dementia diagnosis and subtypes, mental disorders, physical health, anthropometry, demographics, extensive noncommunicable disease risk factor questionnaires, disability/functioning, health service utilization, care arrangements and caregiver strain). The net result is a unique resource of directly comparable data, comprising 21 000 older adults from three continents. An incidence phase was completed in 2010, following up participants 3–5 years after baseline, in China, Cuba, Dominican Republic, Mexico, Peru and Venezuela. This phase of the project included over 12 000 older people and provided in excess of 35 000 person years of follow-up, making it one of the largest-ever studies of the incidence of dementia and associated risk factors. A publicly accessible data archive has been established as a resource for the academic and policy community. Nested within the population-based studies is a randomized controlled trial of a carer intervention for people with dementia and their families – "Helping Carers to Care".

The work of the 10/66 Dementia Research Group is described in detail on the group's web site at http: //www.alz.co.uk/1066/.

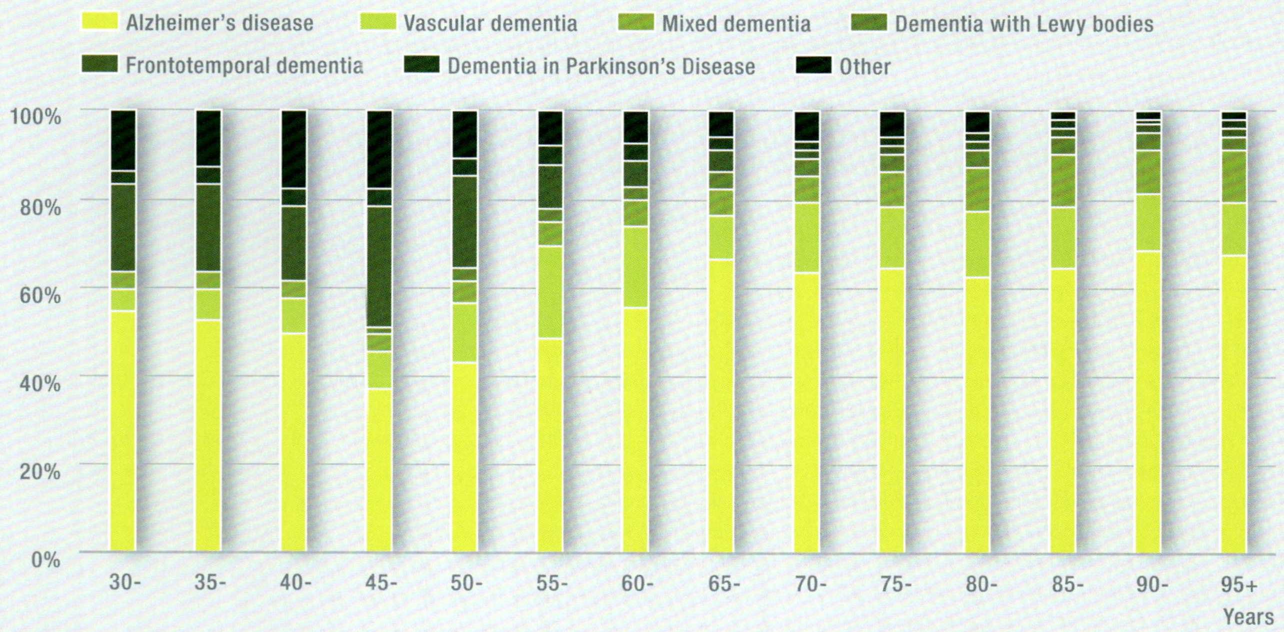


FIG 2.4 A *Dementia UK* report: consensus estimates of the proportion of all dementia cases accounted for by different dementia subtypes, by age and gender. **Women**

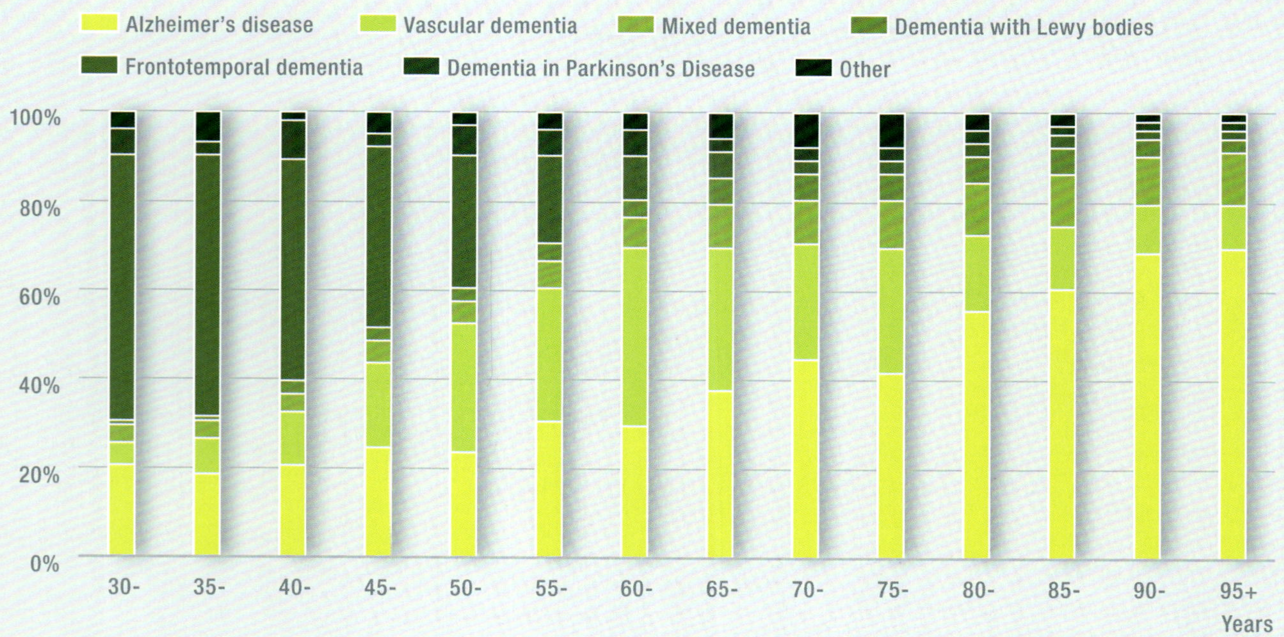


FIG 2.4 B *Dementia UK* report: consensus estimates of the proportion of all dementia cases accounted for by different dementia subtypes, by age and gender. **Men**

(Reproduced with permission from Alzheimer's Society) *Source: Reference 23.*

## GLOBAL INCIDENCE OF DEMENTIA

Studies of the incidence of the Alzheimer's disease subtype were recently systematically reviewed *(55)*. Twenty-seven studies were identified, of which only seven were conducted outside of North American and Europe – three from Japan, and one each from China (Province of Taiwan), India, Nigeria and Brazil. Hence, only three studies were performed in LMIC. Incidence at age 80 was higher in North America (20.6 / 1 000 person years) and Europe (15.1) than in other countries (8.3). However, the doubling time was shorter in other countries (5.0 years) than in North America (6.0) or Europe (5.8). Incidence was slightly higher among women (13.7 per 1 000 person years) than in men (10.6 / 1 000 person years). The last review of the incidence of dementia was conducted in 1998, in which 23 studies were identified, with only one from LMIC *(56)*. Incidence in Europe increased from 9 per 1 000 person years at ages 60–64 to 180 per 1 000 person years at ages 90–94. A new review was conducted to estimate annual incidence rates and expected annual numbers of new cases in 21 GBD regions. Details of the methodology are in the web appendix which can be found at the online appendix[1].

### SEARCH RESULTS

The search yielded 1 718 abstracts, from which we identified 34 fully eligible studies. Of these, 16 had been conducted in Western Europe, five in North America (four in the USA and one in Canada), four in East Asia (four in China, including one in the Province of Taiwan), six in Latin America or the Caribbean (Brazil, Cuba, Dominican Republic, Mexico, Peru and Venezuela), one in Australasia (Australia), one in the Asia Pacific region (Republic of Korea), and one in West sub-Saharan Africa (Nigeria). Details of eligible studies are provided in a online appendix[1]. Collectively, the studies included 72 224 older people "at risk" and accumulated 214 756 person years of follow-up. The median cohort at risk was 1 769 (interquartile range 937–3 208) and the median person years was 4679 (interquartile range 2 795–9 101). Most studies applied DSM-III-R (n=14), DSM-IV (n=14) or ICD-10 (n=3) criteria. The six 10/66 Dementia Research Group studies applied both DSM-IV and 10/66 dementia criteria.

1. http://www.who.int/mental_health/publications/dementia_report_2012

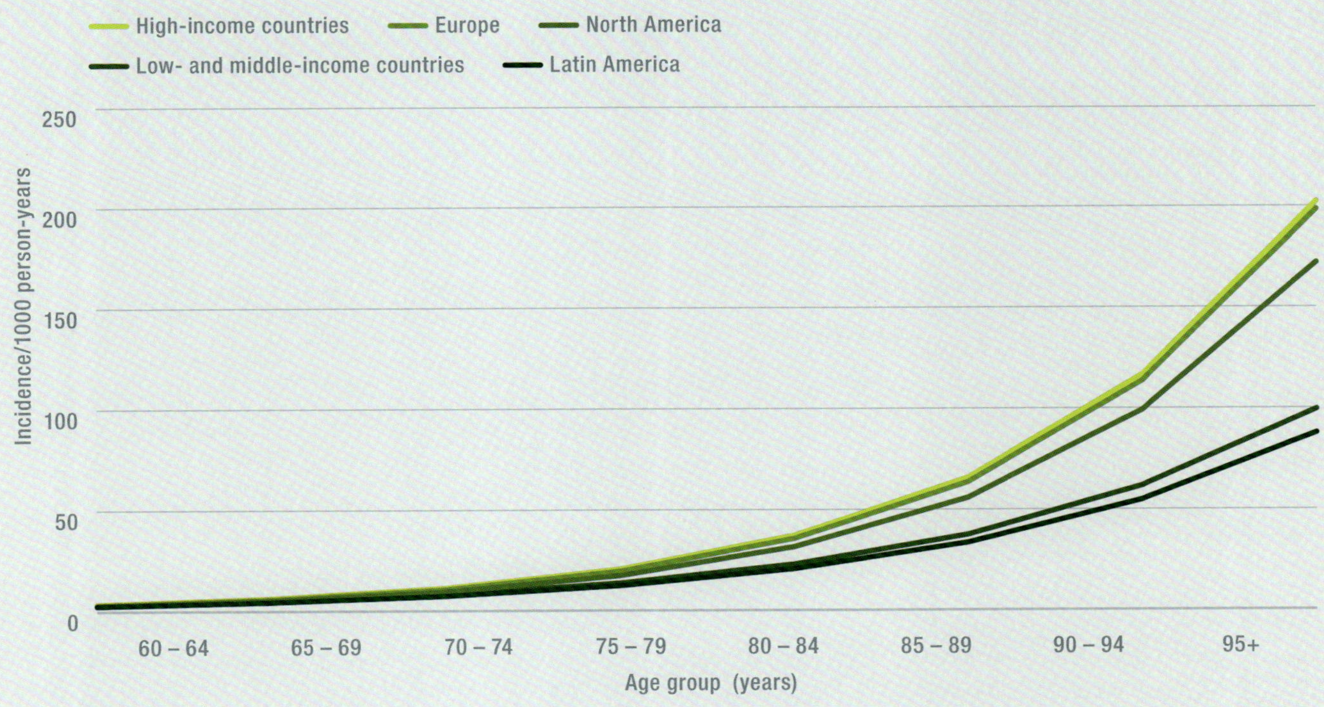


FIG 2.5 Estimated age-specific annual incidence of dementia, derived from mixed-effects Poisson metaregression, for world regions for which meta-analytical synthesis was feasible

| GBD region | Age group (years) | | | | | | | Total |
|---|---|---|---|---|---|---|---|---|
| | 60–64 | 65–69 | 70–74 | 75–79 | 80–84 | 85–89 | 90+ | |
| Australasia | 5015 | 6267 | 8562 | 11718 | 15671 | 15069 | 11999 | 74300 |
| Asia Pacific High Income | 44218 | 60232 | 90569 | 130732 | 156054 | 135777 | 111191 | 728772 |
| Oceania | 689 | 768 | 953 | 922 | 747 | 420 | 275 | 4774 |
| Asia Central | 5426 | 6445 | 13850 | 12735 | 14683 | 7189 | 6031 | 66359 |
| Asia East | 163609 | 191710 | 251150 | 289363 | 249859 | 152360 | 74608 | 1372660 |
| Asia South | 119516 | 151533 | 182288 | 189982 | 155836 | 90384 | 43394 | 932933 |
| Asia Southeast | 47446 | 61200 | 75941 | 80040 | 64702 | 34953 | 13514 | 377795 |
| **ASIA** | **385919** | **478154** | **623312** | **715492** | **657552** | **436153** | **261012** | **3557595** |
| Europe Central | 21552 | 27947 | 46233 | 65949 | 72545 | 51032 | 27739 | 312995 |
| Europe Eastern | 33771 | 40091 | 95946 | 99652 | 137457 | 79242 | 58657 | 544817 |
| Europe Western | 75483 | 114043 | 182382 | 261542 | 332145 | 314136 | 206964 | 1486695 |
| **EUROPE** | **130807** | **182081** | **324561** | **427143** | **542147** | **444410** | **293360** | **2344507** |
| North America High Income | 52406 | 70167 | 94281 | 130578 | 174934 | 173137 | 147305 | 842808 |
| Caribbean | 3979 | 5197 | 6475 | 7178 | 7348 | 4968 | 4405 | 39551 |
| Latin America Andean | 3776 | 4764 | 5908 | 6462 | 5804 | 3624 | 1210 | 31548 |
| Latin America Central | 16610 | 20338 | 24059 | 27602 | 26361 | 18371 | 6392 | 139732 |
| Latin America Southern | 6399 | 8654 | 11164 | 14077 | 14829 | 10133 | 2958 | 68215 |
| Latin America Tropical | 16786 | 20071 | 25269 | 26023 | 24696 | 14745 | 4303 | 131892 |
| **THE AMERICAS** | **99956** | **129191** | **167156** | **211919** | **253972** | **224979** | **166572** | **1253746** |
| North Africa/ Middle East | 30328 | 35742 | 45605 | 50307 | 41393 | 19764 | 9488 | 232627 |
| Sub-Saharan Africa Central | 4019 | 5120 | 5814 | 5602 | 4173 | 2052 | 926 | 27706 |
| Sub-Saharan Africa East | 16318 | 20287 | 23222 | 23251 | 17922 | 9318 | 4636 | 114953 |
| Sub-Saharan Africa Southern | 4461 | 5839 | 6838 | 7150 | 6092 | 3656 | 2429 | 36465 |
| Sub-Saharan Africa West | 15252 | 19618 | 23002 | 22915 | 18614 | 9902 | 4762 | 114067 |
| **AFRICA** | **70378** | **86606** | **104481** | **109225** | **88194** | **44692** | **22247** | **525818** |
| **WORLD TOTAL** | **687060** | **876031** | **1219510** | **1463780** | **1541864** | **1150234** | **743185** | **7681665** |

TABLE 2.4 Estimated annual numbers of incident cases of dementia, by age group and Global Burden of Disease region

## COVERAGE

While the evidence base from Europe and North America dominated, 13 of the 34 studies were from outside these regions, and 10 studies were conducted in countries with low or middle income regions. There was no coverage for nine GBD regions: Oceania, South-East Asia, Central Asia, Central Europe, Eastern Europe, North Africa/Middle East, Southern sub-Saharan Africa, Central sub-Saharan Africa and Eastern sub-Saharan Africa. Five studies (four in Europe and one in the USA) focused on persons aged 80 years or over. The Western European studies contributed 52% of the total person years, the North American studies 21% and the Latin American studies 15%, with just 12% contributed by studies from other regions.

## MODELLING THE INCIDENCE OF DEMENTIA

The incidence of dementia increases exponentially with increasing age. For all studies combined, the incidence of dementia doubles with every 5.9 year increase in age, from 3.1 per 1000 person years at age 60–64 to 175.0 per 1 000 person years at age 95+ (Figure 2.5). The incidence of dementia appears to be higher in countries with high incomes (doubling every 5.8 years from 3.4 per 1 000 person years to 202.2 per 1 000 person years) than in LMIC (doubling every 6.7 years from 2.9 per 1 000 person years to 99.4 per 1 000 person years). Overall the incidence of dementia in LMIC was 36% lower (RR 0.64, 95% CI 0.48–0.85) than in high-income countries. However, if the 10/66 Dementia Research Group's cross-culturally validated 10/66 dementia criteria were applied rather than DSM-IV criteria, then this difference was no longer apparent (RR 0.99, 95% CI 0.74–1.33). There was significant heterogeneity in the incidence estimates when all studies were combined (alpha = 0.16). Heterogeneity was greater for studies in countries with high incomes (0.17) than in countries with low or middle incomes (0.02).

### ESTIMATION OF ANNUAL NUMBERS OF INCIDENT CASES OF DEMENTIA

Numbers of new cases increase and then decline with increasing age in each region; in Europe and the Americas peak incidence is among those aged 80–89 years, in Asia it is among those aged 75–84 years, and in Africa among those aged 70–79 years (Table 2.4). The researchers estimated nearly 7.7 million new cases of dementia each year worldwide, implying one new case every 4 seconds. Some 3.6 million (46%) would impact in Asia, 2.3 million (31%) in Europe, 1.2 million (16%) in the Americas, and 0.5 million (7%) in Africa.

### DISCUSSION – THE INCIDENCE OF DEMENTIA

Incidence rates and numbers of new cases are particularly relevant to efforts to develop, initiate and monitor prevention strategies. Prevalence differences between populations and trends in prevalence over time are difficult to interpret since they may arise from differences in underlying incidence or duration (survival with dementia). The current estimate of 7.7 million new cases per year is an important benchmark, globally and regionally, particularly given the relatively low levels of heterogeneity between studies. Prevalence (35.6 million) is 4.6 times annual incidence, suggesting an approximate average survival from onset of 4.6 years, which is broadly consistent with earlier estimates from case series *(57)*.

Various explanations have been advanced for previous observations of very low prevalences of dementia in some LMIC sites. Estimates of the incidence of dementia were also exceptionally low in the US-Nigeria and US-India studies, suggesting that differences in survival could have been only part of the explanation for the low prevalence recorded in those sites *(58, 59)*. Differences in levels of exposure to environmental risk factors may also have contributed (e.g. the healthy cardiovascular status of older Nigerians) *(60, 61)*. Differing patterns of mortality in early life might also be implicated; older people in very poor countries are exceptional survivors, and some of the factors that confer survival advantage may also protect against dementia onset in late life. However, the evidence from our meta-analysis suggests that differences in dementia incidence between developed and developing countries may not be as large as had previously been suggested, and that methodological factors, particularly the use of DSM-IV diagnostic criteria, may have contributed. For the 10/66 Dementia Research Group studies, as with prevalence *(20)*, the incidence of 10/66 dementia is higher than that of DSM-IV dementia, and when that criterion is applied in this meta-analysis the developed/developing country incidence rates converge. Clearly more research is required into the incidence of dementia in order to provide more evidence on the extent of the problem in different world regions.

## MORTALITY ASSOCIATED WITH DEMENTIA

Dementia shortens the lives of those who develop the condition. One of the best studies in the field estimated median survival with Alzheimer's disease at 7.1 years (95% CI 6.7–7.5 years) and for VaD 3.9 years (3.5–4.2 years) *(57)*. There is much individual variability around these median estimates. The independent contribution of dementia to mortality is difficult to assess. Death certificates are unreliable, since dementia is rarely considered as a direct or underlying cause of death. People with dementia often have comorbid health conditions that may or may not be related to the dementia process and which themselves may hasten death. Hence deaths of people with dementia cannot automatically be considered to be deaths attributable to dementia.

### REVIEW

A meta-analysis of studies principally from high-income countries estimated a two-and-a-half-fold increased mortality risk for people with dementia (RR 2.63, 95% CI 2.17–3.21) *(62)*. The EURODEM incidence studies reported a constant relative risk of 2.38 up to age 89 years, declining to 1.80 in females and 1.60 in males over the age of 90 years. Estimates from LMIC suggest a slightly higher relative mortality hazard: in the 10/66 Dementia Research Group studies, the pooled HR was 2.77 (95% CI 2.47–3.10), with a modest degree of heterogeneity, while even larger relative risks have been recorded in studies in Nigeria (HR 2.83, 95% CI 1.10–7.27) *(63)* and Brazil (HR 5.16, 95% CI 3.74–7.12) *(64)*. In the three studies published to date that have compared dementia with other health and sociodemographic factors influencing mortality in countries with low or middle incomes, dementia emerged as the leading contributor among health conditions *(63–65)*.

In the *Dementia UK* report, the EURODEM mortality relative risks were used to calculate the proportion of deaths at different ages independently attributable to dementia *(26)*. This proportion increased steadily from 2% at age 65 years to a peak of 18% at age 85–89 years in men, and from 1% at age 65 to a peak of 23% at age 85–89 in women. Overall, 10% of deaths in men over 65 years, and 15% of deaths in women are attributable to dementia, the majority occurring among those aged 80–95 years.

Estimates of deaths attributable to dementia from the GBD Report *(6)* are much more conservative – 4.0% of deaths (275 000) among those aged 60 and over in high-income countries, 0.6% (19 000) in upper-middle-income countries, 0.6% (72 000) in lower-middle-income countries and 1.3% (111 000) in lower-income countries, amounting to 477 000 annual deaths worldwide, just 1.6% of the global total for this age group.

# ECONOMIC IMPACT: THE GLOBAL SOCIETAL COST OF DEMENTIA

A proper understanding of the societal costs of dementia, and how these impact upon families, governments and their health and social care systems, is fundamental to raising awareness, achieving proper prioritization, and focusing efforts to improve the lives of people with dementia and their caregivers. Cost-of-illness studies for dementia have been carried out for some, mainly high-income, countries such as Australia *(66)*, Canada *(67)*, Sweden *(68)*, United Kingdom *(26)* and the USA *(69)*, as well as the European Union *(70)*. The consensus is that dementia is already imposing huge economic burdens, both through direct (medical and social care) and indirect costs (unpaid caregiving by families and friends). Evidence is also emerging of the extent of the economic burden in middle-income countries *(71–74)*.

Cost-of-illness studies are descriptive, quantifying the total societal economic burden of a health condition and highlighting its impact on different health and social care sectors. The distribution of costs between countries and regions can also be estimated and compared, and trends over time can be monitored or, tentatively, projected into the future. Comparison of costs of illness across health conditions is more challenging; it has also been argued that prioritization for investment should be determined more by the relative cost-effectiveness of available interventions than by the economic burden of the disease *(75)*.

Three previous reports of the global economic burden of dementia were each based on the best available data for the prevalence of dementia and care inputs *(76–78)*. The most recent of these estimated global costs at US$ 422 billion in 2009, 74% contributed by high-income countries. The aim of this recent cost-of-illness study was to generate evidence-based estimates of resource utilization for each country. Thus, country-specific annual per capita costs (direct medical and social care costs and informal care) were applied to estimated numbers of people with dementia in each country, and aggregated up to the level of WHO regions, and World Bank country income-level groupings. The methodology for estimation of costs is provided in Box 2.2. The costs (as well as the prevalence of dementia) reflect estimates for 2010. Cost estimates based on previous years are inflated appropriately. Costs are expressed as US dollars, converted from local currencies based on current exchange rates. Where no estimates were available for a country, estimates from other similar countries within the same region or adjacent regions were used. For direct costs, the strong relationship between the direct costs per person with dementia and per capita Gross Domestic Product (GDP) was used to predict total direct costs for countries within regions with no data. The split between medical and social care costs was estimated by applying data from China, the one LMIC with available data.

The major limitation was the sparse data on health and social care from LMIC, with cost models relying largely on extrapolation of economic conditions from higher-income to lower-income countries, adjusted for per capita GDP. Also, it was not possible to distinguish between direct medical costs (within the health care sector) and direct social care costs (within the community and care-home sector). The cost of illness analysis conducted for ADI's *World Alzheimer Report 2010 (79)* addressed many of these limitations.

## THE GLOBAL COSTS OF DEMENTIA (BASE CASE OPTION)

The total global societal costs of dementia were US$ 604 billion in 2010 (Table 2.5). This corresponds to 1.0% of the aggregated worldwide GDP, or 0.6% if only direct costs are considered. The total cost as a proportion of GDP varied from 0.24% in low-income countries to 1.24% in high-income countries, with the highest proportions in North America (1.30%) and Western Europe (1.29%). The per capita costs of dementia varied considerably by World Bank income classification, from US$ 868 in low-income countries, to US$ 3109 in lower-middle-income countries, to US$ 6827 in upper-middle-income countries, to US$ 32 865 in high-income countries. When multiplied by the estimated numbers of people with dementia, this generated aggregated costs of US$ 4.37 billion in low-income countries, US$ 29.21 billion in lower-middle-income countries, US$ 32.39 billion in upper-middle-income countries, and US$ 537.91 billion in high-income countries. Therefore, the costs of dementia are unevenly distributed. About 70% of the global societal costs of dementia occur in just two WHO GBD regions (North America and Western Europe) and 89% of the total costs are incurred in high-income countries. However, the minority (46%) of people with dementia live in high-income countries, 39% of people with dementia live in middle-income countries (where 10% of costs are incurred) and 14% in low-income countries (accounting for less than 1% of the total costs).

The distribution of total costs between sectors also varies markedly by country income level. In high-income countries, the costs of informal care (45%) and the direct costs of social care (40%) contribute similar proportions to total costs, while the proportionate contribution of direct medical costs (15%) are much lower (Figure 2.6). However, in low-income countries and lower-middle-income countries direct social care costs are small and informal care costs predominate. Thus, while the total cost per person with dementia is 38 times higher in high-income countries than in low-income countries, the direct costs of social care are 120 times higher. In the ADI worldwide survey of care home utilization, the proportion of people with dementia living in care homes was significantly higher in high-income countries (30%, 95% CI 23–37%) than in LMIC (11%, 95% CI 5–17%).

BOX 2.2

## METHODOLOGY FOR ESTIMATION OF UTILIZATION OF MEDICAL AND SOCIAL CARE, AND INFORMAL CARE

### INSTITUTIONAL CARE

ADI had commissioned a worldwide questionnaire survey of key informants to estimate the proportion of people with dementia residing in care homes, separately for both urban and rural areas. These were merged into a single weighted proportion of people with dementia living in care homes and hence unlikely to be in receipt of informal care.

### INFORMAL CARE

Care inputs by family members, friends and others have an important influence on the societal costs of dementia. The base option was the combined total of basic activities of daily living (ADL, e.g. eating, dressing, bathing, toileting, grooming) and instrumental activities of daily living (IADL, e.g. shopping, preparing food, using transport, and managing personal finances) care inputs. More papers describe combined ADLs than describe only basic ADL care inputs: 42 studies covering 30 countries representing 73% of the worldwide dementia population (average caregiver input 3.6 hours/day [range 1.4–4.7 h/d)]). An opportunity cost approach was used, valuing informal care by the average wage for each country, adjusted for gender differences in average wage for male and female carers.

### DIRECT COSTS

For each country, estimates were sought of both total direct costs and the distribution between direct medical and social care costs. Data on direct costs were available from the country itself or from the region for 95 countries representing 76% of the worldwide dementia population. For the remaining 97 countries, mainly in Africa and Asia, the imputation approach described above was used.

### SENSITIVITY ANALYSIS

Since cost-of-illness studies depend on a set of sources and assumptions, comprehensive sensitivity analyses were conducted to estimate the effect of varying source data or assumptions on cost estimates, as follows:

- the base case use of exchange with purchasing power parity (PPP);
- the types of informal care included in cost estimations;
- the hourly costs to be attached to informal caregiver inputs;
- a replacement cost approach instead of an opportunity cost;
- the relative cost of inputs from different types of caregiver.

### REPRESENTATIVENESS

Of the total of 42 studies that were used for estimating the costs of informal care, 11 studies had population-based designs (cohort studies, case-control studies) or included controls (people without dementia). For the direct costs, the corresponding figures were 11 out of 31 studies. Thus there is still a risk that costs may be overestimated since the results are partly based on non-population-based studies or on studies without controls.

## SENSITIVITY ANALYSES

If only basic ADLs are used for the costs of informal care instead of combining basic ADLs and IADLs, the total costs are 22% lower. They are 30% higher if combined ADLs/IADLs and supervision are included. Compared with US$ 604 billion in the base case, these sensitivity analyses provide a lower bound of US$ 470 billion (only basic ADLs) and an upper bound of US$ 783 billion (all informal care including assistance with basic ADL and IADL and supervision).

Since a substantial proportion of caregivers are spouses and most, but not all, could be assumed to be beyond the usual working age, the informal care and total costs were recalculated by applying a reduced wage to the estimated proportion of caregivers in each country who were spouses. This leads to a 9% reduction in the total worldwide cost estimate from US$ 604 billion to US$ 548 billion when costed at 50% of the average wage and a 14% reduction to US$ 520 billion when costed at 25% of the average wage. With the replacement costs approach, based on the average wage of a social care professional in that country, the total costs were slightly higher.

Under the base case option, low-income countries accounted for just 0.7% of total worldwide costs, middle-income countries for 10.2% and high-income countries for 89.1%. Using PPP rather than exchange rates to translate costs in local currencies to the common US dollar metric, the proportions increased for low-income countries (2.1%) and middle-income countries (20.0%) and fell for high-income countries (77.9%).

| GBD region | Per capita costs (US$) | Number of people with dementia | Aggregated costs (billions US$) | | | | Total costs as % of GDP | Direct costs as % of GDP |
|---|---|---|---|---|---|---|---|---|
| | | | Informal care (all ADLs) | Direct medical costs | Direct Social costs | Total costs | | |
| Australasia | 32 370 | 311 327 | 4.30 | 0.70 | 5.07 | 10.08 | 0.97% | 0.56% |
| Asia Pacific High Income | 29 057 | 2 826 388 | 34.60 | 5.23 | 42.29 | 82.13 | 1.31% | 0.76% |
| Oceania | 6 059 | 16 553 | 0.07 | 0.02 | 0.01 | 0.10 | 0.46% | 0.12% |
| Asia Central | 2 862 | 330 125 | 0.43 | 0.28 | 0.24 | 0.94 | 0.36% | 0.20% |
| Asia East | 4 078 | 5 494 387 | 15.24 | 4.33 | 2.84 | 22.41 | 0.40% | 0.13% |
| Asia South | 903 | 4 475 324 | 2.31 | 1.16 | 0.57 | 4.04 | 0.25% | 0.11% |
| Asia Southeast | 1 601 | 2 482 076 | 1.77 | 1.48 | 0.73 | 3.97 | 0.28% | 0.15% |
| Europe Western | 30 122 | 6 975 540 | 87.05 | 30.19 | 92.88 | 210.12 | 1.29% | 0.75% |
| Europe Central | 12 891 | 1 100 759 | 8.59 | 2.67 | 2.94 | 14.19 | 1.10% | 0.44% |
| Europe Eastern | 7 667 | 1 869 242 | 7.96 | 3.42 | 2.94 | 14.33 | 0.90% | 0.40% |
| North America High Income | 48 605 | 4 383 057 | 78.76 | 36.83 | 97.45 | 213.04 | 1.30% | 0.82% |
| Caribbean | 9 092 | 327 825 | 1.50 | 0.78 | 0.71 | 2.98 | 1.06% | 0.53% |
| Latin America Andean | 3 663 | 254 925 | 0.35 | 0.31 | 0.28 | 0.93 | 0.43% | 0.27% |
| Latin America Central | 5 536 | 1 185 559 | 1.58 | 2.61 | 2.37 | 6.56 | 0.37% | 0.28% |
| Latin America Southern | 8 243 | 614 523 | 2.36 | 1.42 | 1.29 | 5.07 | 1.02% | 0.54% |
| Latin America Tropical | 6 881 | 1 054 560 | 2.17 | 2.67 | 2.42 | 7.26 | 0.42% | 0.29% |
| North Africa / Middle East | 3 296 | 1 145 633 | 1.90 | 2.05 | 0.54 | 4.50 | 0.16% | 0.09% |
| Sub-Saharan Africa Central | 1 081 | 67 775 | 0.04 | 0.02 | 0.01 | 0.07 | 0.06% | 0.02% |
| Sub-Saharan Africa East | 1 122 | 360 602 | 0.28 | 0.08 | 0.04 | 0.40 | 0.17% | 0.05% |
| Sub-Saharan Africa Southern | 6 834 | 100 733 | 0.52 | 0.11 | 0.06 | 0.69 | 0.24% | 0.06% |
| Sub-Saharan Africa West | 969 | 181 803 | 0.11 | 0.04 | 0.02 | 0.18 | 0.06% | 0.02% |
| **World Bank classification** | | | | | | | | |
| Low income | 868 | 5 036 979 | 2.52 | 1.23 | 0.62 | 4.37 | 0.24% | 0.10% |
| Lower middle income | 3 109 | 9 395 204 | 18.90 | 6.74 | 3.57 | 29.21 | 0.35% | 0.12% |
| Upper middle income | 6 827 | 4 759 025 | 13.70 | 10.44 | 8.35 | 32.49 | 0.50% | 0.29% |
| High income | 32 865 | 16 367 508 | 216.77 | 78.00 | 243.14 | 537.91 | 1.24% | 0.74% |
| **Total** | **16 986** | **35 558 717** | **251.89** | **96.41** | **255.69** | **603.99** | **1.01%** | **0.59%** |

TABLE 2.5 Per capita (US$) and aggregated costs (billions US$) by Global Burden of Disease region and World Bank income classification

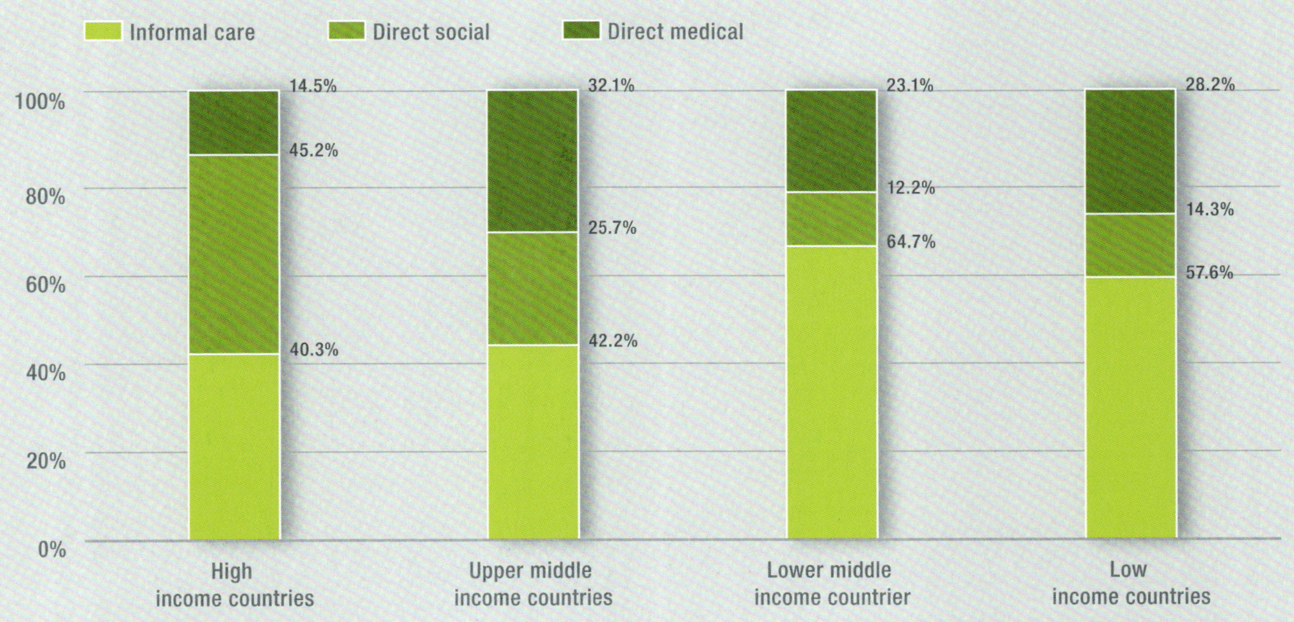


FIG 2.6 Distribution of total societal costs (%) by World Bank Income level

## DISCUSSION – THE ECONOMIC COST OF DEMENTIA

The estimated annual worldwide cost to society of dementia, US$ 604 billion, highlights the enormous impact that dementia has on socioeconomic conditions worldwide. If dementia care were a country, it would be the world's 21st largest economy, ranking between Poland and Saudi Arabia. The scale of these costs is understandable given that:

- the 35.6 million people worldwide comprise 0.5% of the world's total population;
- a high proportion of people with dementia need some care, ranging from support with IADL, to full personal care and round-the-clock supervision;
- in some high-income countries, one third to one half of people with dementia live in resource- and cost-intensive residential or nursing homes *(26, 80)*.

The marked imbalance in the global distribution of prevalence and costs arises, in part, because of the imbalance of costs between sectors. In LMIC, the formal social care sector (accounting for the direct costs of care in the community by paid social care professionals, and of care homes) is practically non-existent. Therefore, responsibility falls largely on unpaid informal caregivers, and informal care costs predominate. In high-income countries the direct costs of social care account for nearly half of all costs. Since average wages (used to estimate informal care costs) are much lower in LMIC, this has an important impact on comparative total costs.

It is difficult to compare our estimates of the global societal costs for dementia with those for other conditions because few such estimates exist and there are problems with comparability. In the United Kingdom, a recent report commissioned by the Alzheimer's Research Trust focused on the economic burden of dementia and other chronic diseases, and sought to compare like-for-like disease costs with national expenditure on research *(81)*. The societal costs of dementia (£23 billion) almost matched those of cancer (£12 billion), heart disease (£8 billion) and stroke (£5 billion) combined. However, for every £1 million in costs arising from the disease, £129 269 was spent on cancer research, £73 153 on heart disease research and £4 882 on dementia research. In a paper from Sweden the costs of dementia were compared with other estimates for chronic disorders *(82)*. The annual costs of dementia (50 billion SEK) was higher than for depression (32.5 billion SEK), stroke (12.5 billion SEK), alcohol abuse (21–30 billion SEK) and osteoporosis (4.6 billion SEK).

# ETIOLOGY AND POTENTIAL FOR PREVENTION

The US National Institutes of Health (NIH) conducted a state-of-the-science conference review in 2010 to provide health-care providers, patients and the public with an assessment of currently available data on prevention of Alzheimer's disease and cognitive decline *(83)*. Their report states that "firm conclusions cannot be drawn about the association of any modifiable risk factor with cognitive decline or Alzheimer's disease". However, the evidence base is still incomplete and further research is required. Very few primary prevention randomized controlled trials have been conducted, and the results do not support potential for risk reduction (see below). Nevertheless, many of these trials recruited older people, and follow-up periods were relatively short. Given that neurodegeneration may precede the onset of dementia by several decades, this may have been a case of too little too late. There is, however, a strong evidence base from population-based cohort studies attesting to the potential risk reduction benefits of better cardiovascular health, more education, and higher levels of physical activity.

### DEMENTIA, CARDIOVASCULAR RISK FACTORS AND CARDIOVASCULAR DISEASE

Research suggests that vascular disease predisposes to Alzheimer's disease as well as to vascular dementia *(84)*. In short *(85–87)* and longer latency *(88, 89)* incidence studies, smoking increases the risk for Alzheimer's disease. Diabetes is also a risk factor *(90)* and, in longer-term cohort studies, midlife hypertension *(91, 92)* and raised cholesterol *(92)* are associated with the onset of Alzheimer's disease in later life. Aggregated cardiovascular risk indices incorporating hypertension, diabetes, hypercholesterolemia and smoking increase risk for dementia incidence incrementally whether exposure is measured in midlife *(89)* or a few years before onset of dementia *(87)*.

Despite occasional negative findings from large prospective studies *(93, 94)*, the accumulated evidence for a causal role for cardiovascular risk factors and cardiovascular disease in the etiology of dementia and Alzheimer's disease is very strong. This has led to speculation that atherosclerosis and Alzheimer's disease are linked disease processes *(95)*, with common pathophysiological and etiologic underpinnings (APOE e4 polymorphism, hypercholesterolemia, hypertension, hyperhomocysteinemia, diabetes, metabolic syndrome, smoking, systemic inflammation, increased fat intake and obesity).

One of the complicating factors for interventions in this area is that evidence suggests that while hypertension, raised cholesterol and obesity in midlife increase the risk for later onset of dementia, blood pressure levels *(91)*, cholesterol *(96)* and body mass index *(97)* fall progressively before the onset of the disease. Hence people with dementia have lower blood pressure levels, cholesterol and body mass than others. Therefore, early primary prevention may be the most effective intervention. Preventive trials indicate that statins *(98)* and antihypertensive treatment *(99)* do not seem to lower the incidence of dementia when initiated in older people, but there have been no long-term trials from midlife onwards.

### EDUCATION AND COGNITIVE RESERVE

Despite some inconsistency among cohort studies, there is quite convincing evidence from high-income countries that higher levels of education and occupational attainment are associated with a lower incidence of dementia *(100)*. Evidence from LMIC is more limited. As roles and responsibilities for older adults vary among cultures, so may the cognitive skills required to maintain them in the face of neurodegeneration; education and occupational attainment may be less relevant in LMIC and less clearly associated with dementia risk. In Beijing, China *(101)* and Cantanduva, Brazil *(14)* there was tentative evidence for a protective effect of literacy. In Brazil, there was also a nonsignificant trend towards lower rates of dementia with higher levels of education *(14)*. Neither study tested for the effect of occupational attainment.

### UNDERACTIVITY

Evidence from epidemiological cohort studies suggests that underactivity is a risk factor for the onset of dementia, and that aerobic exercise may reduce cognitive decline and protect against dementia *(102, 103)*. Meta-analyses of randomized controlled trials of aerobic exercise in healthy adults provide inconsistent but generally positive evidence for cognitive benefits *(103, 104)*. Increased hippocampal volumes, attenuation of age-related grey matter volume loss, and improved neural network connectivity have also been observed *(103)*. Reduced cerebrovascular risk may contribute *(103)*. There have been no randomized controlled trials of the benefit or harm of aerobic exercise for the prevention of dementia.

Following the NIH state-of-the-science review, another group working in the USA conducted systematic reviews into the epidemiological evidence for risk reduction focussing on seven risk factors for which there was strong evidence of independent effects on the incidence of Alzheimer's disease; diabetes, midlife hypertension and obesity, depression, physical inactivity, smoking and low education; assessing evidence pertaining to the USA and populations worldwide *(105)*. Having meta-analysed the evidence base to estimate the relative risk (RR), the reviewers combined this with the prevalence of the risk factor in the population to compute a population attributable risk (PAR) – the proportion of cases of Alzheimer's disease in the population that might be prevented if the risk factor could be removed entirely. From the worldwide perspective, the meta-analysed RR and PAR were as follows: diabetes (RR 1.39, 95% CI 1.17–1.66; PAR 2.4%, 95% CI 1.1–4.1), midlife hypertension (RR 1.61, 95% CI 1.16–2.24; PAR 5.1%, 95% CI 1.4–9.9), midlife obesity (RR 1.60, 95% CI 1.34–1.92; PAR 2.0%, 95% CI 1.1–3.0), depression (RR 1.90, 95% CI 1.55–2.33; PAR 10.6%, 95% CI 6.8–14.9), physical inactivity (RR 1.82, 95% CI 1.19–2.78, PAR 12.7%, 95% CI 3.3–24.0), smoking (RR 1.59, 95% CI 1.15–2.20, PAR 13.9%, 95% CI 3.9–24.7) and low education (RR 1.59, 95% CI 1.35–1.86, PAR 19.1%, 95% CI 12.3–25.6). Thus, the most promising strategies for prevention were the elimination of physical inactivity (12.7% of Alzheimer's disease cases prevented), smoking (13.9% prevented) and low education (19.1% prevented). This is because these factors are both relatively common and strongly associated with Alzheimer's disease. If all the risk factors were eliminated, a total of up to 50.7% of all cases of Alzheimer's disease worldwide might be prevented. Of course, this is implausible. The authors therefore modelled the effect of a more realistic 10% or 25% reduction in the prevalence of the risk exposures on the prevalence of dementia. Using our estimates of 7.7 million new cases of dementia annually, and assuming that the risk reductions would apply to dementia generally and not Alzheimer's disease subtypes alone, we would estimate using the figures provided in the paper that a 10% reduction in exposure to all risk factors could in principle lead to a 250000 (3.3%) reduction in annual numbers of new cases of dementia worldwide, while a 25% reduction in risk factor exposure could prevent 680000 new cases (8.8%) annually.

### DISCUSSION – THE ETIOLOGY AND PREVENTION OF DEMENTIA

There is an underlying assumption in all such calculations that the associations observed in the epidemiological research studies that the risk factor has caused the onset of Alzheimer's disease. This may not necessarily be the case since confounding may have occurred. Other factors associated with, for instance, smoking may have been the true risk factor. In epidemiological studies one tries to adjust for the effect of such confounding variables, but this may not be completely successful. Reverse causality also needs to be considered – i.e. the early pre-clinical effects of Alzheimer's disease neuropathology may include a tendency to be less physically active or to become depressed – and hence the disease may cause the risk factor rather than the risk factor causing the disease. It is for these reasons that policy-makers and advisers (such as the recent NIH state-of-the-science expert panel *(83)*) are reluctant to act on the basis of epidemiological evidence alone. Randomized controlled trials of the effects of removing or reducing the risk factor are considered to provide the best quality of evidence. However, these are difficult to conduct due to the long latency between the period during which the risk factor exerts an influence on the mechanisms that lead to dementia (early age to midlife) and the onset of dementia in late life.

The best hope of ascertaining the likely impact of increasing levels of education and improvements in cardiovascular health may be to observe populations in which such trends are prominent, and to see whether these are associated with a decline over time in the age-specific incidence of dementia. Detection and treatment of diabetes and hypertension, reduction in levels of obesity, smoking cessation, increased physical activity and better education are already public health priorities for most countries worldwide. In comparison with most high-income countries, efforts to prevent and control the coming epidemic of cardiovascular and other chronic diseases in LMIC are in their infancy *(106)*. Advocated measures include implementation of tobacco-free policies, comprehensive bans on advertising and taxation of tobacco products, salt reduction through voluntary agreements with the food industry, and combination drug therapy for those at high risk of cardiovascular disease *(106)*. The detection and control of hypertension, hyperlipidaemia, diabetes and metabolic syndrome is poorly implemented by overstretched primary care services that struggle to cope with the burden of historic priorities (such as maternal and child health, and communicable diseases) and the rising tide of chronic disease in adults. Many health systems are not trained, equipped or structured to deal with the latter. The message that dementia, alongside heart disease, stroke and cancer, may be prevented through increased adoption and more effective implementation of these public health strategies is one that policy-makers and the public need to hear.

## LIMITATIONS

This report assembles, for the first time, global evidence on the incidence as well as the prevalence of dementia, estimates of the prevalence of YOD, the societal economic cost of dementia, and the potential for prevention. This work has benefited from the recent expansion of the evidence base on the prevalence and incidence of dementia, and care inputs in LMIC. It is now possible to rely less on expert opinion guided by scant research, and more on the direct evidence of the accumulated data. These data have corrected an earlier impression that the prevalence of dementia is much lower in developing as compared with developed countries. The extended evidence base, and the detailed estimates provided, while still provisional, constitute the best currently available basis for policy-making, planning and allocation of health, welfare and population prevention resources.

However, there are some limitations to this review. The main ones are the poor coverage of the evidence base in many world regions, the poor quality of some of the studies that were included in the review, and the heterogeneity of estimates between studies within regions. These issues are considered below.

### COVERAGE

The recent expansion of population-based research into dementia in the Caribbean, China and Latin America means that the coverage of the evidence base for these regions is now as good as for North America and Western Europe. However, our reviews highlight continued deficiencies in research evidence. Adequate coverage of large and populous countries such as China or the USA would require many studies in different regions encompassing the racial, cultural, economic and social diversity of the nation as a whole. The best approach would be a survey of a nationally representative sample, but very few examples exist, such as those in Canada *(19)* and in the USA (on a small sample) *(107)*. Studies carried out in just one or two countries may not safely be generalized to a large number of other countries in the same GBD region. Limits to generalizability are particularly marked when the few or only available studies are small, conducted some time ago, and/or of poor methodological quality. The low estimated prevalence in sub-Saharan Africa was greatly influenced by the one good quality study from that continent *(16)*. The North Africa and Middle Eastern region includes as many older people as the whole of sub-Saharan Africa, and with a much steeper projected increase in numbers. As yet, only one study from Egypt *(22)* and one from Turkey *(108)* were eligible for inclusion in the review. Central Asia and Eastern Europe (including Russia) remain essentially uncovered by research and estimates remain highly tentative. South-East Asia is represented by five studies, but there are none from Indonesia whose 21 million older people account for two-fifths of the total for the whole region.

The evidence base for the incidence of dementia is not as extensive as that for the prevalence of dementia. There is good coverage for Europe, but there are relatively few North American studies. The recently completed 10/66 Dementia Research Group studies have improved coverage in China and Latin America. However, East Asia is still represented by just four studies, with no evidence at all for South Asia or South-East Asia. The continent of Africa is represented by just one study. Therefore, despite minimal heterogeneity between studies included in this review, there is continuing uncertainty as to the true incidence in LMIC and whether, as has been suggested previously with respect to Alzheimer's disease *(55, 109, 110)*, the incidence may be much lower in some developing regions than in other higher-income regions.

The cost-of-illness analyses presented in this report are based on better underlying sources than previous worldwide estimates but there are significant limitations. Studies of dementia prevalence and dementia-related resource utilization are unequally distributed worldwide, with data lacking from many countries. Even with the recent increase in population surveys conducted in LMIC there is a particular lack of studies from Africa, Eastern Europe and the Middle East. Data on resource utilization is also more extensive than previously, particularly with respect to informal care provision in LMIC. The 10/66 Dementia Research Group studies in China, India and Latin America *(3, 111)* add significantly to the pre-existing database, which was heavily skewed to European and North American studies. The results from the ADI worldwide survey of key informants regarding placement in residential care is also a great advance from previous studies.

An important finding of this review has been that descriptive population-based research into dementia in high-income countries peaked in the 1990s and has declined sharply since then. Prevalence can change over time, either because of changes in disease incidence (e.g. because of improvements in cardiovascular health) or disease duration (e.g. reductions in dementia mortality associated with improved long-term care). Future policy-making and planning requires accurate up-to-date figures, and these are no longer available for most high-income countries. Such studies, should ideally be repeated using similar methodology in order to track secular trends in the prevalence and incidence of dementia and in service utilization.

## QUALITY

The quality of prevalence studies is a cause for concern since the problems identified can all lead to biased and inaccurate estimates of prevalence and numbers. Dementia diagnosis requires a multidomain cognitive test battery, an informant interview, a structured disability assessment and a clinical interview to exclude other causes of cognitive impairment, yet fewer than half of all studies met these standards, with the informant interview most frequently omitted. The effect of inadequate ascertainment procedures on dementia prevalence is uncertain. The misapplication of study designs involving two or more phases was widespread. The correct procedures for designing, conducting and analysing such studies are well established *(112)*. However, awareness among dementia researchers remains limited. Misapplication of multiphase methods will always tend towards an underestimation of true dementia prevalence and an overestimation of precision. Multiphase studies are also complicated by the often quite high levels of loss to follow-up that occur between the screening and definitive diagnostic assessment *(17)*. This is again likely to lead to bias which could be towards overestimation or underestimation of true prevalence *(113)*.

With respect to the economic analyses, it should be noted that most resource utilization studies have been carried out on "convenience samples" of persons who have accessed services (rather than representative population-based studies) and are hence skewed towards those with greater needs for care, which may result in an overestimate of costs. The LMIC estimates of informal care were based largely on the 10/66 population-based studies in China, India and Latin America *(111, 114)* where in most study sites some 30–50% of those with dementia were rated as needing "no care", while most high-income country estimates are derived from convenience samples. This may have led to a systematic overestimate of costs in high-income countries settings. However, many of the resource utilization studies from high-income countries were conducted in the 1990s, since when the uptake of formal health and social care services may have increased.

## HETEROGENEITY

A fundamental assumption, implicit in the modelling approach in this review, was that the prevalence and incidence of dementia were uniform within GBD regions and that they could be estimated from the available evidence and applied to all countries a particular region. In fact, contrary to some previous suggestions *(115)*, statistically significant heterogeneity of prevalence and incidence was in almost all regions. This is not surprising given the varied languages, cultures, levels of development and demographic compositions of the national and subnational units that make up a GBD world region. Methodological variability can be reduced through standardization of study procedures. The way in which the diagnosis of dementia is defined and applied may be among the most important sources of variability. The use of DSM-IV criteria, the most widely applied dementia diagnosis, is not fully operationalized, although it can be *(116)*. An international consensus regarding what constitutes cognitive impairment, what constitutes social and occupational impairment, and how these should be measured would be desirable. Specific research diagnostic criteria would therefore be helpful, with due allowance made for cultural differences. Recent proposals for development of ICD-11 and DSM-V may meet some of these requirements *(117, 118)*.

# FUTURE TRENDS

The reported projections for future growth in numbers of people with dementia should be treated with caution. First, these rely on demographic projections which may not be accurate for many parts of the world, especially for older age groups. Second, it was assumed that age-specific prevalence in each region would remain constant over time. However, changes in risk exposure may increase or decrease incidence. Conversely specific therapies and better social and medical care may reduce case mortality and increase prevalence. Disease-modifying therapies that delay onset, even to a modest extent, would have considerable potential for reducing age-specific prevalence.

It is particularly difficult to make confident projections of future economic costs. If we assume that all potential background factors remain unchanged, and we factor in only the forecast increases in the number of people with dementia, then by 2030 worldwide societal costs will have increased by 85%. The reality is more complicated. Future costs could be influenced by macroeconomic factors (e.g. the pace of economic development) and by dementia-specific factors. These would include changes in the prevalence of dementia, in patterns of help-seeking and trends towards earlier diagnosis, in the availability of health and social care services, changes in care systems and care conditions and the availability of new and more effective treatments. There are very few estimates of the extent of the "treatment gap" for dementia in LMIC, but it is likely to be much greater than in better-resourced settings *(119)*. The current inequitable distribution in dementia costs between world regions will also have implications for future trends, which are likely to tend towards more rapidly increasing per capita and population costs in LMIC, with the result that the global distribution of costs will come to resemble that of morbidity. These cost increases will be driven by several underlying factors. First, increases in numbers of people with dementia will occur much more rapidly in LMIC because of the more rapid demographic ageing in those regions. Second, with economic development, wages will rise rather rapidly in LMIC. Third, resources for dementia care, particularly formal medical and social care, are unequally distributed worldwide. With increased awareness will come increased demand for care. Residential and community social care systems are well developed in many high-income countries but are scarce in LMIC where there is a reliance on traditional, informal family care arrangements. In many LMIC the traditional family and kinship structures are under threat from the demographic, social and economic changes that accompany economic development and globalization. Therefore, the need for community and residential care is likely to grow in LMIC, and with it direct costs.

# SUMMARY POINTS

- It is estimated that in 2010 there were 35.6 million people living with dementia, with 7.7 million new cases each year.
- Numbers of people with dementia will nearly double every 20 years, with much of the increase occurring in rapidly developing middle-income countries. Currently, 58% of people with dementia live in LMIC, and this proportion is projected to rise to 71% by 2050.
- Dementia onsets are rare before the age of 65 years but are likely to be under-ascertained, with young onset dementia accounting for 2–9% of all cases.
- The global societal economic cost of dementia is US$ 604 billion, of which 89% is incurred in high-income countries.
- In high-income countries, numbers of people with dementia will continue to increase, particularly among the oldest old. The provision and financing of their long-term care needs, including support for their family carers, will inevitably become an increasingly urgent political priority.
- If patterns of morbidity and mortality in LMIC converge with those of high-income countries, then dementia prevalence levels will do likewise. The implication is that the projections of rates of growth in the numbers of people with dementia in LMIC, and associated costs (based on an assumption of constant prevalence), may be conservative.
- Informal care costs predominate in LMIC, where institutionalization is uncommon and where community services are poorly developed.
- Efforts to improve the quality and availability of care, and to seek for cure, should be coupled with urgent investment in primary prevention measures. More research is required to identify modifiable risk factors.
- Primary prevention should focus on targets suggested by current evidence, namely: improving access to education and countering risk factors for vascular disease, including diabetes, midlife hypertension, midlife obesity, smoking, and physical inactivity.
- The progress of the dementia epidemic must be monitored in all world regions, with assessment of the effectiveness of prevention programmes and the impact of measures taken to increase the coverage of care. The current evidence base provides a strong baseline which will be improved as evidence accumulates from currently underrepresented regions.

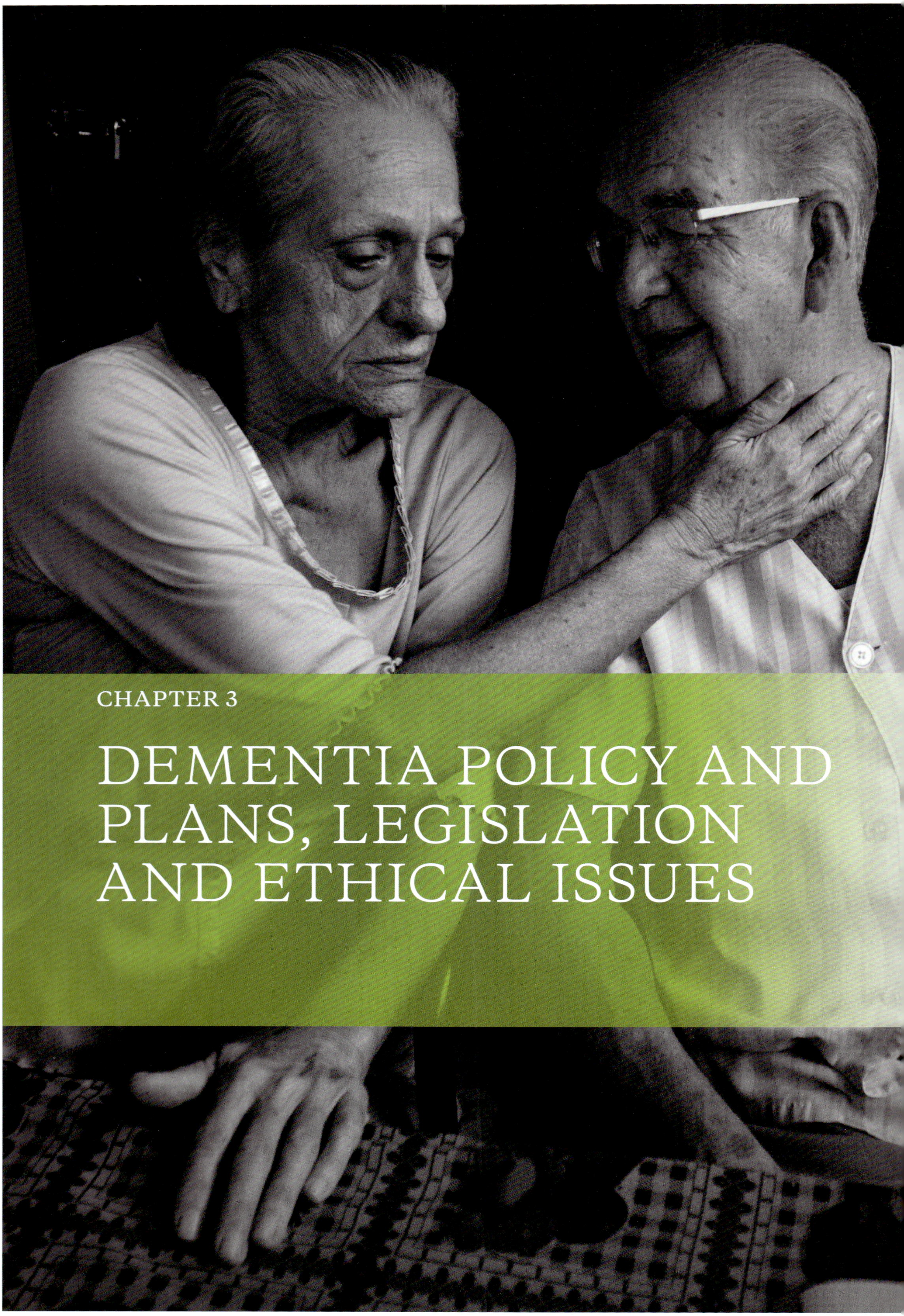

CHAPTER 3

# DEMENTIA POLICY AND PLANS, LEGISLATION AND ETHICAL ISSUES

Given the huge burden of dementia on people with dementia and their caregivers, the challenges facing governments worldwide are substantial. The last decade has seen a growing recognition of the scale of the problem and the need for action. Some countries have developed dementia strategies, policies, plans or guidelines. Common elements include: the need for a coordinated multisectoral approach; the need to provide accessible, affordable and good quality health and social care and services that meet the needs and expectations of people with dementia and their families; and the importance of ethical, social, legal and financial protection. For LMIC countries, there is the opportunity not to repeat the mistakes of high-income countries that have become over-dependent on costly institutional care.

This chapter gives an overview of some national responses to dementia. It includes a brief report of countries with formal plans and other countries that have taken significant steps towards addressing many of the aspects relating to a public health approach to dementia. The content of dementia policies, plan and strategies, and the level of detail differ from country to country. However, each provides information that can be shared and lessons learned. As WHO's Director-General, Dr Chan, has stated, "As health systems are highly context-specific, there is no single set of best practices that can be put forward as a model for improved performance. But health systems that function well have certain shared characteristics" *(120)*. This overview provides the basis for a description of key aspects when developing national dementia policies, plans or strategies.

The chapter also reviews social and financial support systems and legislative structures, highlighting the need for promotion of human rights and protection from abuse and loss of freedoms when capacity and independence become compromised. Finally, the chapter highlights the need for ethical decision-making at every level of response to dementia, including planning, service provision and day-by-day support for people with dementia and their families.

# DEMENTIA POLICIES, PLANS AND STRATEGIES

## NATIONAL AND SUBNATIONAL DEMENTIA POLICIES AND PLANS

Countries use diverse approaches to improve the quality of life of people with dementia and their caregivers. Some have launched policies, others plans, strategies or frameworks. There is considerable variability in how countries use these terms. The present report uses the term "policy and/or plan" for any government policy document, plan or strategy in which a framework for action is articulated. However, when referencing to a particular official document from a particular country, the exact terminology used in the document is retained. For example, England has a strategy "Living well with dementia: A National Dementia Strategy" *(121)*.

Table 3.1 provides a brief overview of the policies/plans/strategies – including the objective, key areas for action, and the time frame for implementation of the plan. For further details, please refer to the source documents.

In addition, several other countries – such as China, Czech Republic, India, Malta, Northern Ireland and the USA – are currently developing national approaches to respond to the impact of dementia. However, these have not yet been finalized or implemented *(137, 138)*. Other countries in Europe have identified dementia as a priority and have initiated steps towards the development of a national dementia policy or plan – such as Belgium, Cyprus, Finland, Luxembourg, Portugal and Switzerland. Sweden in 1992 developed a social policy on dementia arguing for a "normalization process" – i.e. even if you have dementia, you should live a normal life, similar to that of all citizens in the community *(139)* – marking a radical change over previous theories. In 2010 Sweden also presented specified national guidelines for dementia care *(140)*. Germany does not have a national dementia plan but the issue of dementia is considered a priority and addressed through various Ministries (Health, Family, Seniors, Research, Work and Social Affairs) *(138)*. In some countries, state or regional policies have been or are being developed because the country takes a decentralized approach to health and social care – as in Australia, Canada, Switzerland and the USA.

## CIVIL SOCIETY INITIATIVES

ADI, an international federation of Alzheimer associations around the world, released the Kyoto Declaration in 2004 *(141)* providing minimum recommendations for dementia care based on overall recommendations from WHO's World health report 2001 which focused on mental health *(142)*. Recognizing that countries are at different levels of resource development, it proposes a feasible, pragmatic series of objectives and actions for health systems at all levels of development. It defines responses to each of the 10 actions at three levels of attainment: for countries with low, medium and high levels of resources (Box 3.1).

In 2006 Alzheimer Europe adopted a declaration on the political priorities of the European Alzheimer Movement *(143)*. The Paris Declaration calls on European national policy-makers to give Alzheimer's disease and other forms of dementia the political priority they deserve. The declaration covers public health, research, health (medical) care, social support, and legal and ethical priorities. In many of the countries described in Table 3.1, Alzheimer associations have been key partners or stakeholders in the development and/or implementation of national or subnational policies/plans/strategies.

| Country | Policy/plan/ strategy title | Vision/aim/objectives | Areas of actions | Timeline | Source |
|---|---|---|---|---|---|
| **Australia** | *The Dementia Initiative: Making Dementia a National Health Priority* | "A better quality of life for people living with dementia and their carers and families" | • Community care packages<br>• Training for aged care staff<br>• Dementia Behaviour Management Advisory Service<br>• Support and information for individuals with dementia and families<br>• Research funding<br>• Community support grants | 2005–2011 Funding continuing to 2013 | *Reference 122* |
| **Canada (Subnational plan in Ontario)** | *Alzheimer Strategy – Preparing for our future* | "To support people with dementia and their carers, through the implementation of three measures" | • Staff education and training<br>• Physician training<br>• Increased public awareness, information and education<br>• Planning for appropriate, safe and secure environments<br>• Respite services for caregivers<br>• Research on caregiver needs<br>• Advance directives on care choices<br>• Psychogeriatric consulting resources<br>• Coordinated specialized diagnosis and support<br>• Intergenerational volunteer initiative | 1999–2004 | *Reference 123* |
| **Denmark** | *National Dementia Action Plan* | – | The plan has 14 recommendations focused around:<br>• timely diagnosis<br>• quality in diagnosis<br>• improved interdisciplinary communication<br>• care for people with dementia and their informal caregivers<br>• awareness, particularly of advanced care planning and preparing future caregivers | 2011–2015 | *Reference 124* |
| **England** | *Living well with dementia: A National Dementia Strategy* | "For people with dementia and their family carers to be helped to live well with dementia, no matter what the stage of their illness or where they are in the health and social care system' | The strategy has 17 recommendations, comprising three main themes:<br>• Raising awareness and understanding<br>• Early diagnosis and support<br>• Develop services to assist people in living well with dementia | 2009–2014 | *Reference 121* |
| **France** | *French Alzheimer's Disease Plan* | • To improve the quality of life for people with dementia and their caregivers<br>• To develop our understanding of the disease for future action<br>• To mobilise society for the fight against dementia | • Increasing support for caregivers<br>• Strengthening coordination between all actors involved<br>• Enabling patients and their families to choose support at home<br>• Improving access to diagnosis and care pathways<br>• Improving residential care for better quality of life for Alzheimer's Disease sufferers<br>• Recognising skills and developing training for health professionals<br>• Making unprecedented efforts in research<br>• Organising epidemiological surveillance and follow up<br>• Providing information for general public awareness<br>• Promoting ethical considerations and an ethical approach<br>• Making Alzheimer's Disease a European priority | 2008–2012 | *Reference 125* |
| **Japan** | *Emergency Project for Improvement of Medical Care and Quality of Life for People with Dementia* | "To build a society, where people can live life safely without anxiety even after being affected by dementia, where they can be supported by appropriate and integrated services of medical care, long-term care and community care" | • Investigation of situation<br>• Acceleration of the research and development<br>• Promotion of early diagnosis and provision of appropriate medical care<br>• Dissemination of adequate care and support<br>• Measures for people with early-onset dementia | 2008 (no end date) | *References 126 and 127* |
| **Korea (Republic of)** | *War on Dementia* | Dementia is a national health care priority | 2008–2010:<br>• Early diagnosis<br>• Prevention and treatment<br>• Infrastructure building<br>• Public awareness<br><br>2011–2013:<br>• Expand outreach service<br>• Upgrade long-term care insurance<br>• Dementia Service Network<br>• Managing Dementia Law | 2008–2013 | *References 128 and 129* |

**TABLE 3.1** National and subnational dementia policies and plans

Note: Plans in publication as of January 2012

| Country | Policy / plan / strategy title | Vision / aim / objectives | Areas of actions | Timeline | Source |
|---|---|---|---|---|---|
| **Netherlands** | Caring for people with dementia | "To improve the quality of life of people with dementia and their carers; and to provide professionals with the tools they need to care effectively" | • Creating a coordinated range of care options that meet the client's needs and wishes<br>• Sufficient guidance and support for people with dementia and their caregivers<br>• Measuring quality with dementia care indicators<br>• The key outcome should be to secure the continuum of care. | 2008–2011 | *Reference 130* |
| **Northern Ireland** | *Improving Dementia Services in Northern Ireland* | "To improve the quality of life of people with dementia and their carers; and to provide professionals with the tools they need to care effectively." | • Reducing the risk or delaying the onset of dementia<br>• Raising awareness<br>• Promoting early assessment and diagnosis<br>• Supporting people with dementia<br>• Supporting caregivers<br>• Legislation<br>• Research | 2011–2015 | *Reference 131* |
| **Norway** | *Dementia Plan 2015* | "To improve the care for persons with dementia, the family carers and professional caregivers" | • Improving the quality of care through development measures and research<br>• Raising knowledge / skills of workforce and increasing numbers<br>• Improving collaboration between professions<br>• Support "active care", such as day-care programmes<br>• Support partnership between families and professionals | 2007–2015 | *Reference 132* |
| **Scotland** | *Scotland's National Dementia Strategy* | "Deliver world-class dementia care and treatment in Scotland, ensuring that people with dementia and their families are supported in the best way possible to live well with dementia" | Focusing on two key service delivery areas:<br>• Improved post-diagnostic information and support<br>• Care in general hospitals, including alternatives to admission | 2010–2013, with annual progress reports and a commitment to review plan by 2013 | *Reference 133* |
| **Switzerland** (Subnational plan in Canton of Vaud) | Maladie d'Alzheimer et maladies apparentées | Improve lives of persons with dementia and health care recognition of their needs | • Geriatric assessment and formation/education of medical and health professionals<br>• Care coordination<br>• Respite for family caregivers | 2010–2013 | *Reference 134* |
| **United States of America** (Subnational plans) | Subnational plans (Arkansas, California, Colorado, Illinois, Iowa, Kentucky, Louisiana, Maryland, Michigan, Minnesota, Mississippi, Missouri, New York, North Dakota, Oklahoma, South Carolina, Tennessee, Texas, Vermont, Virginia, West Virginia) | – | The common themes of access to diagnosis, training for professionals and support for family caregivers are central in these plans as is a focus on detection and access to accurate diagnosis | – | *Reference 135* |
| **Wales** | *National Dementia Vision for Wales* | Vision is to create "dementia supportive communities" | • Improving service provision (collaboration)<br>• Early diagnosis and timely interventions<br>• Improving access to information, support, and advocacy services<br>• Improving training for a workforce | 2011 (no end date) | *Reference 136* |

Note: Plans in publication as of January 2012

**BOX 3.1**

## THE ALZHEIMER'S DISEASE INTERNATIONAL KYOTO DECLARATION 2004

**10 AREAS FOR ACTION:**

- Provide treatment in primary care.
- Make appropriate treatments available.
- Give care in the community.
- Educate the public.
- Involve communities, families and consumers.
- Establish national policies, programs and legislation.
- Develop human resources.
- Link with other sectors.
- Monitor community health.
- Support more research.

*Source: Reference 141.*

## DEVELOPING DEMENTIA POLICIES AND PLANS: KEY ASPECTS

As described in Table 3.1, there are several key aspects relating to development and implementation that are common to many of the national dementia policies and plans, and it may be necessary to consider the key aspects as summarized below, to ensure that the policies and plans address needs in an effective and sustainable manner.

### SCOPING THE PROBLEM

At global level the World Alzheimer Reports *(3, 7)* and this report from WHO provide quantification of the extent of the growing impact of dementia on countries. Several countries have developed their own reports on the national prevalence and economic impact of dementia. Before countries develop their national policies or plans, information on population needs such as prevalence and community understanding is required. An evaluation of current health, social and community systems and services, including caregiver support services, and an identification of gaps should also be undertaken. Scoping the problem helps in defining the vision and objectives of the policy and/or plan, and includes the following analysis:

**a) The national numbers** – There is no substitute for reliable national estimates of need, starting with the numbers of persons with dementia. Advances in research into case definition and population-based surveys have yielded solid information on the epidemiology of dementia. This can be used along with local and national demographic data to generate an accurate estimate of the number of people with dementia both in the country and in each region. There is no more powerful tool for obtaining political and financial commitment than locally derived and relevant data.

**b) The national costs** – A primary concern of government is cost. The best available national measures of service use in dementia, plus the costs of services and the numbers of people with dementia can show the costs of dementia. Costing the work done by family caregivers is difficult, and the status of work forgone in order to provide care (opportunity costs) is controversial. A pragmatic approach making the best of data is needed.

**c) Future projections of numbers and cost** – All countries have population projections. The numbers of persons with dementia in the next 20–30 years can also be predicted, as discussed in chapter 2. Reliable estimates of the current situation will allow for the calculation of projections of the growth in numbers and costs of dementia in the future. These figures will make clear the need for a strategic plan for dementia and will strongly support the argument that this should be at national rather than local level.

**d) The state of current services** – If there are high-quality diagnostic, treatment and care services for people with dementia and their families, such services must be preserved and expanded. If, however, services are not "fit for purpose", there may be a need for change. A critical analysis of current service provision, including its strengths and weaknesses, can inform discussion on what a revised system might look like and can be the basis for building that system. Such analyses generally show that the level of diagnosis and treatment of people with dementia is low with high variation between the most active and least active areas.

**e) External validation** – To gain credibility, it is very useful if dispassionate external assessment can come to the same conclusions as the analysis. For instance, in the United Kingdom the work of the National Audit Office *(144)* and the subsequent enquiry by the House of Commons' Public Accounts Committee *(145)* provided vital external validation of the nature and content of the national policy.

### INVOLVING ALL RELEVANT STAKEHOLDERS

Broad consultation with the relevant parties is essential as it can generate a shared understanding and ownership of policy and helps to ensure that strategies address the needs of the dementia community. This process may be time-consuming and labour-intensive, but its potential value is that the inclusiveness and comprehensiveness of the consultation process lend it validity when moving to implementation. In many countries, care of older people with dementia is not the responsibility solely of the Ministry of Health. It also falls under the purview of other ministries such as that responsible for social welfare. Therefore any dementia policy or plan in a country requires coordinated efforts by different government ministries (Box 3.2). Consultations must include health care providers, caregivers and people with dementia. The consultation process should include groups with special needs – including, where appropriate, indigenous and minority ethnic populations, migrant groups, and younger people with dementia.

BOX 3.2

## ORGANIZING DEMENTIA CARE IN LEBANON

Issues related to the welfare of the older population in Lebanon rest primarily with two ministries – the Ministry of Social Affairs and the Ministry of Public Health. In 1999, following the recommendations of the first International Conference on Ageing in Vienna, a National Commission on Ageing was established as an advisory or consultative body to the Minister of Social Affairs who is the commission's Chair. The commission brings together policy-makers from most ministries that have a bearing on issues related to the older people. The commission also includes representatives from civil society associations that provide services to the older people, persons from academia and, more recently, the private sector.

Both the Ministry of Social Affairs and the Ministry of Public Health recognize dementia as a chronic debilitating disease.

Historically, the role of both ministries was to offer partial financial support to people admitted to nursing homes. Civil society organizations, charities and religious associations have been assuming a prominent role in caring for the older people. Recently, however, both ministries became aware that more needs to be done. The Ministry of Public Health provides coverage for some medications and the Ministry of Social Affairs promotes the establishment of adult day-care and "senior clubs" in its dispensaries throughout Lebanon.

*Source: Reference 146.*

BOX 3.3

## FRANCE: NATIONAL PLAN FOR "ALZHEIMER AND RELATED DISEASES"

The French "National plan for 'Alzheimer and related diseases' 2008–2012" demonstrates strong political commitment both to the persons with Alzheimer's and related diseases and their families. The plan pledged 1.6 billion Euros over this period. Its aim is to build a personalized pathway for each patient, from diagnosis to care at home, and in institutions where appropriate. The strategy consists of 44 measurable objectives. Its implementation and assessment processes are available on www.plan-alzheimer.gouv.fr.

Persons with Alzheimer's and related diseases and their caregivers are the main focus of the strategy which has three main priorities:

- making unprecedented efforts in research to find or validate a diagnosis or treatment;
- changing the way dementia is viewed by making it a focus at local, national and international levels;
- improving the quality of life of patients and their families by:
  - promoting timely and accompanied diagnosis everywhere in France; and
  - strengthening, and making more consistent, care and support for patients and their families.

A number of solutions are focused particularly on preventing behavioural and psychological symptoms and delaying loss of autonomy. The strategy aims to provide 500 Alzheimer mobile multidisciplinary teams by the end of 2012. These teams are composed of professionals trained in rehabilitation, stimulation and support of patients and their families.

The French national plan has also expanded the dementia research capacity of France, established new memory clinics and diagnostic centres, and reduced the use of antipsychotic drugs. There is a recognized need to follow this plan with another when it reaches its completion in 2012.

*Source: Reference 125.*

### IDENTIFYING PRIORITY AREAS FOR ACTION

The priority areas should address the key areas identified by the situation analysis. Key areas could include awareness-raising in the community, access to health and social care throughout the course of the illness, development of a skilled health and social support network, support for informal caregivers, and research into prevention and treatment. An overarching principle when developing dementia policies, plans or programmes is to incorporate an ethical approach (this is discussed in detail in a later section). For example, Box 3.3 provides brief information on the priorities identified in the French National Plan.

In the WHO dementia survey, respondents from 12 countries stated that their country provided at least one programme targeting dementia. The most frequently identified programme areas were research (11 countries; 37% of the total) and awareness-raising (10 countries; 33%). For example, both Japan and the Republic of Korea have recognized a need to educate citizens to overcome the stigma and discrimination associated with dementia (Box 6.1 for a summary of Japan's public awareness programme). Risk reduction programmes (8 countries; 27%), community care services (8 countries; 27%), residential care (7 countries; 23%), and education and training for the workforce (7 countries; 23%) were also identified as important areas of action. Respondents from four (13%) countries reported other programmes such as improving management of people with dementia in emergency departments and training in management of behavioural and psychological symptoms of dementia.

### IMPLEMENTING THE POLICY AND PLAN

Implementation can be challenging. Decisions on what to invest in may lie at local level or with independent health care providers. Convincing health planners that investing in dementia services is worthwhile is the focus of the implementation phase. Implementation requires leadership at local, regional and national levels.

### COMMITTING RESOURCES

The financial commitment to the policy and plan is crucial. Funding must be sustainable and reliable. As an example, the Republic of Korea clearly outlines its funding strategy. An increase in health insurance premiums for everyone over the age of 20 will generate funds for services for people over the age of 65 with an ageing-related illness such as dementia. However, it is estimated that only 4% of the older population will be able to receive this government assistance due to a cap on participation rates, while 8.3% of the same population have dementia *(128)*.

### INTERSECTORAL COLLABORATION

In order to ensure maximum benefits, intersectoral collaboration is essential. In addition, the policy and plan should identify the roles and responsibilities of different sectors such as government agencies (health, education, social welfare, housing), academic institutions, professional associations, general health care providers and specialists, dementia advocacy groups, and other NGOs.

### DEVELOPING A TIME FRAME AND A MONITORING AND EVALUATION SYSTEM

Finally, an action plan and a time frame should be developed for each of the areas of action. In addition, the mechanisms for monitoring and evaluating the policy and plan should be explicitly recognized and developed.

### ADDITIONAL CONSIDERATIONS IN LOW- AND MIDDLE-INCOME COUNTRIES

LMIC have a unique set of obstacles to overcome when developing an effective dementia policy and plan.

**Low priority of mental and neurological disorders:** Mental and neurological disorders are often a low priority. The WHO Mental health atlas reported that 60% of countries have a dedicated mental health policy, and 71% possess a mental health plan *(147)*. In most of these countries, there is a specific provision made for the care of persons with dementia. Nigeria has a declaration, but not a formal policy, on ageing. While no specific reference is made to dementia, it is stated that the government regards the care of elderly persons as being of paramount importance *(148)*. In India, there is movement towards special provisions for people with dementia in the National Policy for Older People, and the National Mental Health Programme (Box 3.4).

**Poor awareness and understanding:** This is often a major issue. More attention, commitment and resources are required for raising awareness and improving dementia literacy. People's knowledge and beliefs regarding dementia can vary greatly across cultures and must be considered when developing awareness-raising campaigns (see Chapter 6).

**Lack of infrastructure and resources:** In many LMIC, the health infrastructure is poorly resourced and the primary focus of governments and health providers is communicable diseases. There is an absence of resources for providing effective diagnostic and management processes. The development of services needs to be adaptable to the existing system. Chapter 4 discusses some mechanisms for improving the delivery of dementia services through strengthening health and social care systems.

In addition, many LMIC lack a welfare system, which can result in a significant financial burden for people with dementia and their caregivers. Furthermore, governments are likely to have limited resources to allocate to action on dementia. Sustainable strategies will need to be low-cost in implementation and maintenance, and yet be capable of reaching widespread populations.

Most research into risk factors is conducted in high-income countries. While some risk factors may be applicable globally, more studies in LMIC are needed to better understand the different social and environmental contexts (see Chapter 2 for further details).

**BOX 3.4**

## INDIA: TOWARDS A NATIONAL DEMENTIA POLICY

India is undergoing a demographic transition and conditions related to ageing such as dementia are on the rise. However, awareness is poor, and there is a lot of stigma associated with the symptoms of dementia.

The *Dementia India Report 2010* by the Alzheimer's and Related Disorders Society of India, was released on 21 September 2010 (World Alzheimer's Day). It estimated that that the numbers of people with dementia in India is 3.7 million and this number is set to double in the next 20 years. The report made evidence-based information available in order to help develop a national policy for people with dementia.

The Government of India has begun to realize the extent of the situation and the need to establish dementia-sensitive services. The next few years will see the establishment of the National Institute of Ageing, and special provisions for people with dementia in the National Policy for Older People and the National Mental Health Programme.

In addition, under the Ministry of Social Justice and Empowerment and in the nongovernmental sector, several institutes for home nursing and training programmes in dementia care have been started.

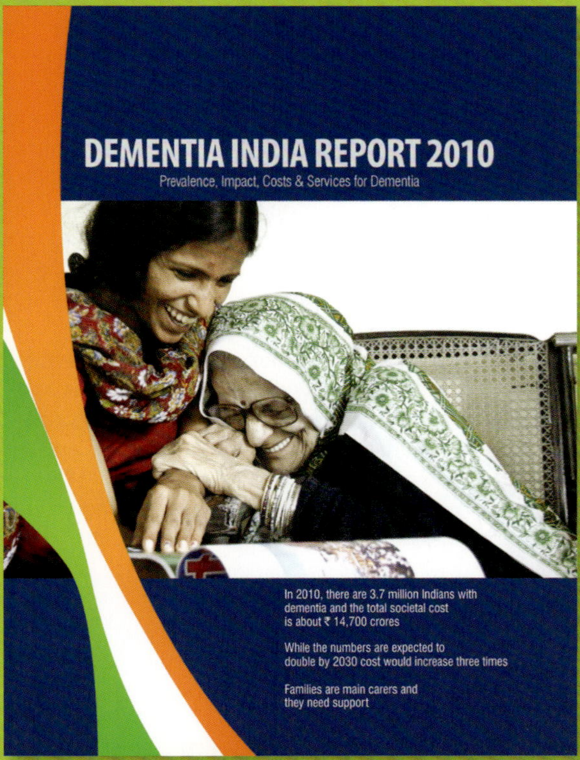


*Source: Reference 149.*

**Linking dementia care with other priorities:** In LMIC, there could be opportunities for integrating dementia care into other policies or priorities (resulting in enhanced dementia care), such as:

- integration of mental health in primary care;
- implementation of WHO's Mental Health Gap Action Programme (mhGAP) with the objective of scaling up care for mental, neurological and substance use disorders (including dementia) in LMIC (Box 4.2);
- implementation of the United Nations' Political Declaration of the High-level Meeting of the General Assembly on the Prevention and Control of Non-communicable Diseases;
- development and implementation of policies and plans for older people;
- proposals for active ageing, especially those that contribute to risk reduction, such as exercise programmes and increasing opportunities for social engagement (Box 6.4);
- improvement of daily living conditions, as recommended by the 2008 WHO Commission on the Social Determinants of Health *(150)*.

# SOCIAL AND LEGAL PROTECTION, HUMAN RIGHTS AND ETHICS

## SOCIAL PROTECTION OF PEOPLE WITH DEMENTIA AND THEIR CAREGIVERS

"There is no subject of greater importance than the ageing of the population and the provision of social protection for older people. It affects the very nature of our societies and concerns not only older people, but all sections of the population" (Joseph Stiglitz, Nobel Prize-winning economist) *(151)*.

### ROLE OF SOCIAL PROTECTION

Social protection is essential to improving access to services and ensuring that people do not experience financial hardship as a result of paying for them. Social protection strategies consist of policies and programmes designed to reduce poverty and people's vulnerability. This is especially important in the current situation of economic slowdown, globalization of diseases, and growing demands for long-term care that is linked, in large part, to ageing populations.

Social protection in old age is fragile and depends on the interaction of many factors – such as health, living arrangements, family support, and sources and levels of income. Some support is available through financial benefits for older people, particularly in high-income countries. However, many people in LMIC cannot access financial benefits such as aged or retirement benefits, disability pension or compensatory benefits for caregivers, and have to rely on out-of-pocket payments for health care and other essential services. This leads to barriers to the access to services for the poor and may result in severe financial difficulties. In low-income countries, the share of out-of-pocket payments in total health expenditure measured in US$ was 50% compared to only 14% in high-income countries (Figure 3.1) *(152)*. Box 3.5 presents a profile of dependence (needs for care) among older people and its consequences in Dominican Republic where pension coverage has been among the lowest in Latin America. In many African and Asian countries, financial barriers and lack of social protection are also prominent, as is evident from the case examples from China and Nigeria (Box 3.5).

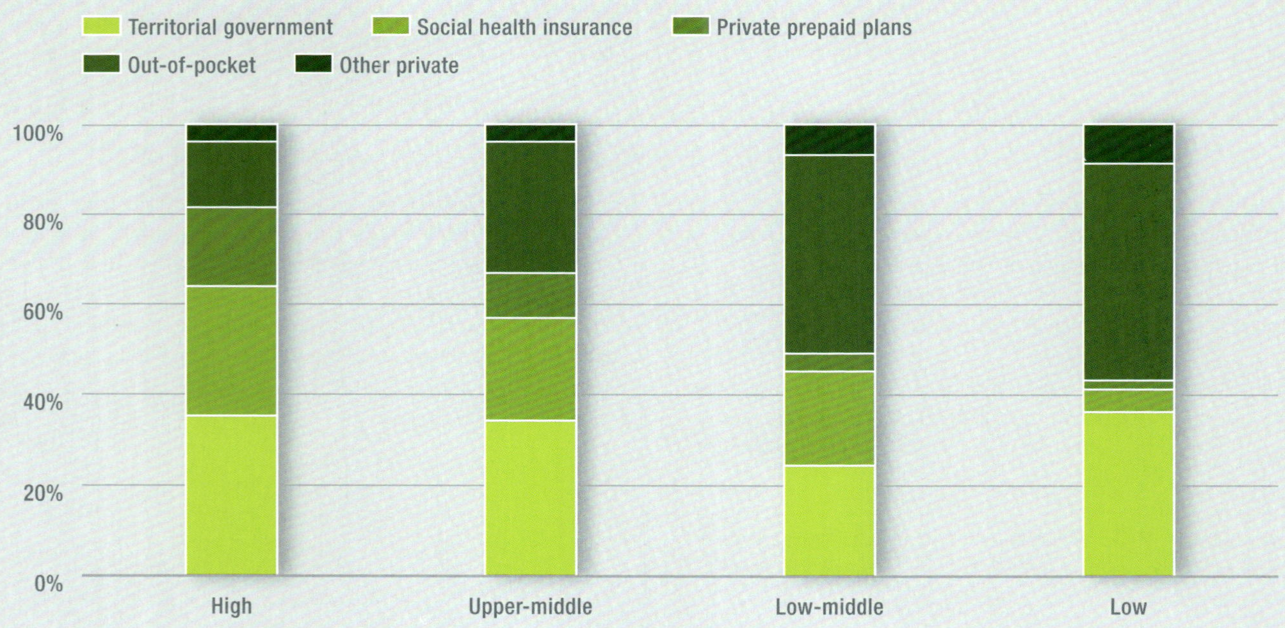


**FIG 3.1** Composition of health expenditure measured in US$. *Source: Reference 152.*

**BOX 3.5**

## INADEQUACY OF SOCIAL PROTECTION

### THE CASE OF THE DOMINICAN REPUBLIC

The Dominican Republic has a population of 9.4 million, of whom 0.5 million (5.7%) are aged 65 and over. Life expectancy is 71 years for men and 75 for women. The Dominican Republic is one of the poorest countries of Latin America, with a per capita GDP of US$ 9200. In common with other countries in the region, the Dominican Republic has high levels of income inequality. Some 42% of the population lives below the poverty line and one third of these are in extreme poverty.

Pension coverage, at only 18% of the economically active population, is one of the lowest in Latin America. Extensive reforms have been proposed, and are in the process of implementation. Community health care is provided by the government through the system of "primary attention units". Consultations are free, but medicines must be paid for. Despite low medical insurance coverage, private health care is widely used. The Dominican Republic has only 20 psychiatrists, 20 psychologists, and two neurologists per million people.

The 10/66 data show that the age standardized prevalence of dependence (needs for care) is nearly as high as in the USA, and dependent older people are less likely to have a pension, much less likely to have paid work, and no more likely to benefit from financial support from their families. Dementia makes the strongest independent contribution to dependence.

*Source: Reference 153.*

### THE CASE OF NIGERIA

Nigeria has the largest population in Africa, with more than 140 million people of whom 3% are aged 65 years and older. Life expectancy is 46 years for men and 47 years for women. It is one of the world's poorest nations, with 90% of the population living on less than US$ 2 per day.

Traditional medicine is widely used. Pension schemes are contributory, and given low literacy and high unemployment rates, pension coverage is low. Disability benefits are available only to people injured in the course of their paid employment.

The 10/66 data show:

- The prevalence of dependence was 24.3%, with a concentration in participants aged 80 and older.
- Only 1% of participants received a pension, and fewer than 7% had paid work.
- Those who were dependent were less likely than others to receive income from their family.

*Source: Reference 148.*

### THE CASE OF CHINA

In the People's Republic of China, financing, coverage and access to health care depend largely on where one lives. Only 61% of rural residents, compared with 82% of urban dwellers, can access health services within one kilometer of their homes. In urban China, there are two employee-based health insurance schemes, one for government employees and the other for public and private company employees. There is limited cover for dependents, based on a personal annual subscription. Discounts are available for poor people, those with mental disorders, and retirees.

In rural China, the government contributes to a common fund which covers health care costs but the government contribution is proportionate to the amount contributed by the employees. In 2003, 79% of rural and 45% of urban residents did not have meaningful health insurance. Almost 50% of health care costs are covered by out-of-pockets payments.

More than 35% of urban and 45% of rural households cannot afford any health care. Social protection (encompassing the range of formal and informal mechanisms to provide safety nets and support to poor and disadvantaged members of society) is under threat for older people in China as the country's population ages rapidly. Among traditional groups in society, social protection is provided by the family and community. However, in the future there will be fewer children available to provide support and care because of the one-child policy.

In summary, the urban bias of public policy is particularly marked in China, and older people living in rural areas may be especially vulnerable. The Research Agenda on Ageing Project has advocated more research on this group, including demographic and migration patterns, social transitions, family exchanges, health behaviors, and use of and access to health care.

*Sources: References 154–156.*

| Population-based catchment area | Number | Receiving a government or occupational pension % | Receiving a disability pension % | Receiving income from family transfers % | Experiencing food insecurity % | No children within 50 miles % |
|---|---|---|---|---|---|---|
| Cuba (urban) | 323 | 81.4 | 0.9 | 7.4 | 5.6 | 19.5 |
| Dominican Republic (urban) | 242 | 27.3 | 0.8 | 23.6 | 13.7 | 25.1 |
| Venezuela (urban) | 146 | 41.1 | 4.1 | 2.7 | 2.7 | 13.4 |
| Peru (urban) | 130 | 58.5 | 1.1 | 5.4 | 1.6 | 16.4 |
| Peru (rural) | 36 | 66.7 | 0.0 | 0.0 | 8.6 | 25.1 |
| Mexico (urban) | 93 | 78.5 | 1.1 | 7.5 | 3.2 | 4.3 |
| Mexico (rural) | 87 | 34.5 | 2.3 | 17.2 | 12.6 | 5.8 |
| China (urban) | 84 | 84.5 | 0.0 | 11.9 | 0.0 | 0.0 |
| China (rural) | 56 | 10.7 | 0.0 | 23.2 | 3.6 | 7.8 |
| India (urban) | 75 | 13.3 | 2.7 | 28.0 | 28.0 | 5.3 |
| India (rural) | 108 | 26.9 | 0.0 | 44.4 | 17.6 | 10.9 |

**TABLE 3.2** Social protection for older people with dementia in LMIC *(158)*

## SOCIAL PROTECTION OF PEOPLE WITH DEMENTIA AND THEIR CAREGIVERS: CURRENT SITUATION

In recent years, high-income countries have seen fiscal challenges for governments in meeting the anticipated spiralling costs of health and long-term social care for older people with chronic diseases, including, and most particularly, dementia. There is also a considerable cost incurred by families, due to caregivers cutting back on paid work, and the high cost of care services where these are not subsidized by the state. In LMIC, despite a greater reliance on the family unit as a resource, family support is neither ubiquitous nor comprehensive. Traditional forms of support are being undermined by greater internal and international migration, declining fertility, higher levels of education and the increased participation of women in the workforce which reduces the availability and willingness of children (principally daughters and daughters-in-law) to provide care *(111)*.

Much of the information from LMIC comes from the 10/66 dementia population-based study centres. A key finding is the economic disadvantage associated with caregiving A high proportion of caregivers had to stop or cut back on pa d work in order to provide care. Few older persons with dementia ir 10/66 LMIC country sites received government or occupational pensions, and virtually none received disability pensions. Alarmingly, high rates of food insecurity (people with dementia going hungry through lack of resources to purchase food) were seen in the Dominican Republic, rural Mexico and rural Peru, and in both Indian sites *(157, 158)*. Gifts of money from family (family transfers) were identified as an important source of income in the 10/66 study centres that have low pension coverage. However, in many of the sites, a substantial minority of the older people with dementia did not have children living locally and available to provide support (Table 3.2).

In some LMIC, governments have sought to place responsibility for the financial support and care of older parents firmly upon families *(111)*. For example, the Indian parliament passed a law in 2007 requiring children to support their parents, with those who fail to do so facing a fine or brief prison term. The law was passed in response to concerns that older persons are being neglected both physically and financially by family members. The legislation also provided for the state to set up old-age homes, access being limited to the poor and the childless. Such legislation is likely to be only partially effective in extending and deepening social protection. Given the demographic, social and economic trends described above, an increasing role for the state seems inevitable (see also Chapter 2). This trend may be managed most effectively by incentivizing and supporting informal family care.

The WHO dementia survey provided additional information on financial benefits for elderly people with dementia and their families. When asked to report on social and financial benefits for people living with dementia, significant differences emerged between responses from high-income countries and LMIC. For example, 19 of 22 (86%) LMIC reported that there was no pension for people with dementia (Figure 3.2). However, Russia reported that when medico-social personnel document the presence of disability in a patient, the patient can receive financial benefits equivalent to about US$ 20 per month. Many survey respondents suggested that people with dementia should receive a disability pension.

All eight high-income countries in the WHO dementia survey reported having a medication subsidy or reimbursement scheme which would apply to medications to improve the symptoms of dementia; however, this may not cover all available medications. Only 6 of 22 (27%) LMIC reported having a medication subsidy scheme. Mexico reported that some medication schemes are available to employees of private companies.

### TOWARDS UNIVERSAL SOCIAL SUPPORT

Health and social care financing based on direct or out-of-pocket payments are particularly problematic for dementia and other chronic diseases in older people. Chronicity implies the need for continuing care, leading to mounting costs. At the same time, older people, particularly in LMIC, tend not to have secure incomes, and families may be experiencing economic strain due to the costs and demands of caring. Universal noncontributory social pensions, targeted disability pensions and caregiver benefits may each have an important role to play in addressing this problem. Social pensions provide insurance against the risks that older people face, including uncertainty over how long they will live, how long they will remain healthy, and whether they can count on the support of others if they need it. Social pensions play a significant role in alleviating chronic poverty *(159)*, as having a pensioner in the family reduces the risk of the household poverty *(160)*. Dependent older persons are particularly likely to benefit as informal care would be bolstered and incentivized, and formal/paid care would be more affordable.

Another mechanism to provide support could be a prepayment approach. When formulating risk-pooling or prepayment approaches, there are three broad issues to be considered. First, pools that protect the health needs of a small number of people are not viable in the long term. Second, in every country there will be a proportion of poor people who will need to be subsidized by the government. Third, contribution must be compulsory for otherwise the rich and healthy will opt out and there will be insufficient funding to cover the needs of the poor and sick *(161)*. An example of a prepayment approach to support those who are facing the need for care as they age is the long-term care insurance in Japan which enables service users to access to a range of services, and not just health services (Box 3.6).

## LEGAL PROTECTION OF PEOPLE WITH DEMENTIA AND THEIR CAREGIVERS

### PROTECTING THE HUMAN RIGHTS OF PEOPLE WITH DEMENTIA

People with dementia and their caregivers have the same human rights as every other citizen.

The United Nations' *Convention on the Rights of Persons with Disabilities* places a general obligation on states to ensure and promote the full realization of all human rights and fundamental freedoms for all persons with disabilities through appropriate legislation, by promoting standards and guidelines, promoting research, providing accessible information, and through promoting the training of relevant professionals and staff in the rights recognized in the convention *(163)*.

In Article 1 of the convention, governments are required to "promote, protect and ensure the full and equal enjoyment of all human rights and fundamental freedoms by all persons with disabilities, and to promote respect for their inherent dignity" *(163, 164)*.

It is widely recognized that people with dementia are frequently denied the basic rights and freedoms available to others. In many countries physical and chemical restraints are used extensively in aged-care facilities and acute-care settings, even when regulations are in place to uphold the rights of people to freedom and choice. The majority of people who are restrained have cognitive impairment *(165)*. The use of restraint is frequently rationalized by those who initiate its use as necessary to ensure the safety of persons restrained, to control agitation and "unacceptable" behaviour, or to prevent interference with or resistance to treatment *(165, 166)*. Such

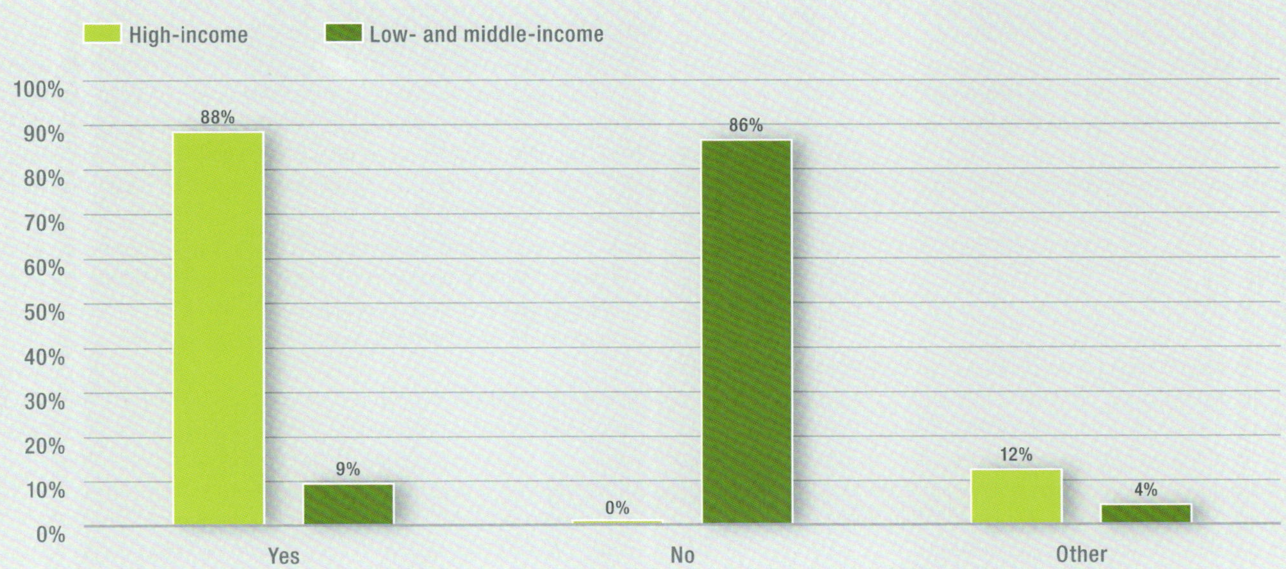


FIG 3.2 WHO dementia survey: Percentage of countries reporting availability of social/financial benefits for people with dementia

attitudes reflect the ethical challenges inherent in the support and protection of people with dementia, and legislation alone will not always ensure the protection of rights. Other deprivations of basic rights may be more willful in intent, such as when a third party uses deceit to acquire access to a person's assets.

It is essential that rights are recognized, respected and protected in order to empower people with dementia, those who support them and the community as a whole. An appropriate and supportive legislative environment is also required to ensure the highest quality of service provision to people with dementia and their caregivers. Fundamental to upholding a person's rights is the recognition of capacity in persons with dementia. Where capacity is impaired due to dementia, a legitimate expectation of the law is that it should establish a structure within which appropriate autonomy and self-determination are recognized and protected.

### PRESENCE OF LEGAL PROVISIONS

In many countries, there exist legal provisions for people whose capacity is impaired due to a mental health condition. These provisions include processes relating to giving or withholding consent to treatment, substitute or supported decision-making, and procedures for implementing advance directives.

The results of a survey carried out in 2005 by Alzheimer Europe provides information on legal approaches to consent, capacity and incapacity in over 20 European countries *(167)*. The legal systems in the responding countries recognized the right of an individual with capacity to give or withhold consent to treatment, and all were based on the presumption of capacity (i.e. persons are assumed to have capacity to make their own decisions unless the opposite has been demonstrated). Most countries had explicit provision for some form of substitute decision-making, primarily through relatives or court-appointed guardians. In some countries, the legislation allowed for a degree of flexibility in these systems, recognizing that capacity may fluctuate or decline over time. A minority of countries have also passed legislation to permit a person to nominate his/her own decision-maker should capacity become impaired in the future, rather than relying on a court decision.

An important component of substitute decision-making is to ensure that the person's rights are protected from abuse or exploitation by a third party or substitute decision-maker. For instance, there should be a process to protect against the misuse of a person's financial assets.

The data collected through the WHO dementia survey suggest that legislation relating to the protection of the rights of elderly people with dementia in LMIC is limited. Table 3.3 from the WHO dementia survey shows the percentage of high-income countries and LMIC which reported on the presence of specific legislation and/or regulation relating to capacity, decision-making and protection against social or financial neglect or abuse.

### CAPACITY AND SUPPORTED DECISION-MAKING

It is a matter of principle that adults who are capable of doing so are entitled to make their own decisions about their health care and personal welfare. The CRPD recognizes that, in cases of disability, people may require support with decision-making. Such a structure should include appropriate supported decision-making processes, in accordance with Article 12.3 of the CRPD which provides that "States Parties shall take appropriate measures to provide access by persons with disabilities to the support they may require in exercising their legal capacity". The question of capacity, however, is not always straightforward in the context of dementia. When can a person who has dementia make informed decisions? Due to the progressive nature of the syndrome, there is the likelihood that the ability to understand and to make informed decisions will be increasingly impaired over time. However, the presence of dementia should not be justification for assuming a person cannot make decisions in all aspects of his/her life.

Article 12 of the CRPD supports a move away from an assumption that people with mental disabilities are incapable of making decisions to a "presumption of capacity" – i.e. a person is assumed to have capacity to make his/her own decisions unless the opposite has been demonstrated in all aspects of decision-making. The convention takes a functional approach to legal capacity, whereby a person's functional abilities, behaviours or capacities (i.e. what a person understands, knows and believes) is directly relevant to the person's ability to make a decision. This is in contrast to the status approach (i.e. a presumption that lack of capacity applies to all people with dementia) or an outcomes-based approach (i.e. evidence of failure in one area implies a lack of capacity in all) *(164)*. While the CRPD relates to people with mental disabilities more generally, it has some application for capacity and decision-making for people with dementia.

To avoid, or at least reduce, the problems inherent in borderline capacity, greater emphasis should be put on supported decision-making – for instance, with trusted family members or a formal advocate. This form of supported decision-making may help bridge the gap between the time when a person with dementia is fully able to make decisions and the time when formal proxy decision-making becomes necessary on a regular basis *(168)*. Even if the support is close to 100%, it should take into account known past preferences *(164)*. A supported decision-making model which involves the person as much as possible at every stage helps to ensure that, when capacity is eventually dramatically impaired, those that have been supporting the person to make decisions over time have a good understanding of the person's preferences and wishes and are thus in a much better position to determine what the person would have wanted.

Article 12.4 of the CRPD outlines effective safeguards to "ensure that measures relating to the exercise of legal capacity respect the rights, will and preferences of the person, are free of conflict of interest and undue influence, are proportional and tailored to the person's circumstances, apply for the shortest time possible and are subject to regular review by a competent, independent and impartial authority or judicial body" *(163)*. In some countries, such as Canada and Sweden, there are examples of supported decision-making models that are being implemented for people with mental disabilities *(169, 170)*.

BOX 3.6

## LONG-TERM CARE INSURANCE IN JAPAN

With the world's highest ageing rate, Japan established the public long-term care insurance system in April 2000. The insurance aims to: support those who are facing the need for long-term care; clarify the relationship between benefits and burdens by way of introducing a social insurance approach; enable service users to receive comprehensive services from a variety of facilities of their choice; and separate long-term care from coverage of health care insurance.

Insurers are primarily municipalities. The insurance is financed from public funds – government and prefectures (37.5%), municipalities (12.5%) – and premiums of the insured (50%). Persons over 40 years of age pay monthly premiums according to their age, income and the area in which they live. The average premium paid per month is 4 160 JPY (approximately US$ 54). When citizens require services covered by the long-term care insurance, they are certified and classified into one of seven eligibility levels by the local certification committee. Standards for certification are uniformly and objectively determined nationwide. The insurance covers 90% of the service charge and users pay the rest out-of-pocket. The insurance covers both ambulatory (e.g. day-care, home visit, short stay) and residential (e.g. intensive care homes) services, including "community-based long-term care services" such as group homes and small-scale multifunctional in-home care services which are designed to support users to remain in their familiar environments. Care managers assist with planning and organizing services and supervise and evaluate the care process as well.

Since 2000, the number of users of long-term care services covered by the insurance, including outreach care in particular, has doubled. The long-term care insurance system has now become indispensable in supporting people, including people over the age of 40 years with dementia, in need of long-term care.

*Source: Reference 162.*

| Legislation and/or regulatory structure: | High-income countries N=8 | LMIC N=22 |
|---|---|---|
| To determine the capacity of a person with dementia to make financial and legal decisions | 7 (87.5%) | 8 (36.3%) |
| To enable supported decision-making when a person may require support in making decisions due to dementia | 6 (75.0%) | 3 (13.6%) |
| To include safeguards protecting from misuse of guardianship and substitute decision-making processes | 6 (75.0%) | 8 (36.3%) |
| To enable the implementation of advanced health care directives (e.g. decisions relating to life-prolonging treatment and life-support measures in the terminal stage of dementia) | 6 (75.0%) | 3 (13.6%) |
| To protect the rights of people against discrimination on the basis of dementia (e.g. relating to employment, accommodation or insurance) | 5 (62.5%) | 4 (18.1%) |
| To protect people with dementia against physical, verbal, financial or emotional neglect or abuse (by family members or service providers or others) | 7 (87.5%) | 6 (27.2%) |

TABLE 3.3 WHO dementia survey: Reported presence of relevant legislation

Early diagnosis also has a potential legal benefit as there is greater likelihood of the person having the capacity to make decisions relating to future financial, medical and lifestyle matters, including, for instance, advance health planning directives. Advance planning is the process of documenting preferences relating to lifestyle and or medical decisions (advanced health directives) while a person has capacity in order that these wishes can be enacted on the person's behalf, should he or she lose capacity. Advance planning may include wishes relating to consent to or refusal of medical treatment or other aspects of care.

## ADDRESSING ETHICAL ISSUES

Consideration of ethical issues in relation to dementia care may often focus on "big" issues such as refusal of treatment and end-of-life decision-making. While these are important, there are many other difficult ethical issues that arise for those involved in ordinary day-to-day care and that are often neglected *(171–174)*. Moreover, cultural differences relevant to care can also become a focus for ethical concerns.

Ethical issues that may require a broad societal approach *(168)* can be briefly described as:

- **Combating stigma:** This will involve implementing strategies to improve public awareness and understanding of dementia, and ensuring that the work of caregivers is properly valued. It will also involve ensuring that dementia, and people with dementia, are accepted and are visible part of society.

- **Resources:** Society has a duty to ensure that all people with dementia, including those with inadequate resources of their own, receive good care. All societies should have mechanisms in place by which its citizens can access such care when needed.

- **Inclusion of people with dementia in everyday society:** People with dementia have the right to live in the community and to have access to health, social and other support services that enable them to lead full and meaningful lives within society. Societies should enable them to take part in activities, have equitable access to facilities and be invo ved in communal life.

- **Research:** If the incidence of dementia is to be reduced, and the lives of people with dementia are to be improved, research is crucial. It is important not only that funding is available but also that mechanisms are in place, including consent procedures that assist appropriate recruitment of people with dementia into research studies.

Ethical issues arise across the trajectory of the person's life with dementia, often starting with the diagnosis *(168, 171, 172)*. There is currently wide variability in the attitudes of health professionals to communicating the diagnosis. They include assumptions about the person's ability to understand and/or to retain the information, concern about the psychological impact, and therapeutic nihilism *(175)*.

An ethical process for communicating the diagnosis would:

- take into account the person's level of understanding, biography, beliefs, psychological condition and wish to know;

- take into account the family structure and level of involvement in the patient's care;

- address uncertainties in the diagnosis;

- provide opportunities for the discussion of options for treatment and support, as well as future planning, including financial, legal and advance health care planning;

- provide opportunity for follow-up, including psychological support as necessary *(176)*.

Numerous ethical issues may arise, some of them in day-to-day care and others at crucial times in the course of dementia. These issues include, but are by no means limited to:

- balancing the confidentiality of the person concerned with informing family members (e.g. with regard to diagnosis);

- balancing a person's previous views and values with current ones, including the role of supported decision-making (as discussed in the section on legislative support);

- balancing safety and freedom;

- use of assistive technologies (often a balance between safety and privacy);

- end-of-life decision-making, such as withholding and withdrawing life-prolonging treatment and palliative care, in the absence of an advance directive.

### APPLICATION OF ETHICAL PRINCIPLES TO DEMENTIA CARE

Ethical principles need to be interpreted in their application to specific situations and individuals, and different principles may need to be integrated or balanced in order to make a decision. They also must be tailored to context *(177, 178)*.

Guidelines can play an important role in enabling care to be delivered to high ethical standards but they need to be interpreted flexibly and sensitively in specific situations. Since an understanding of ethical issues is extremely important, health professionals who work with people with dementia should receive training in ethics just as they need training in other aspects of good dementia care. Such training should address:

- awareness of ethical issues (recognizing that there is an ethical aspect to a decision or care plan);

- principles and perspectives, (understanding the main relevant ethical principles and having an awareness of the differing perspectives of those who may be involved in dementia care);

- knowledge of guidelines and laws (making ethical decisions with knowledge of the relevant guidelines and laws);

- application of principles, guidelines and laws to specific situations;

- support for people with dementia, their families and nonprofessional care workers (knowing how to support them in the ethical aspects of the care they give).

In view of these considerations, possible steps could be to:

- develop ethically appropriate standards of dementia care based on international human rights standards, including the United Nations' *Convention on the Rights of Persons with Disabilities;*

- provide a clear strategy and mechanisms for achieving these standards;

- create a legal framework and guidelines addressing prevention of abuse, processes of decision-making, end-of-life care, and people's rights;

- provide training on human rights for professional clinicians involved in the support of people with dementia, including family caregivers (such training should address the ethical issues that arise in dementia care, including how to provide support to nonprofessional caregivers in coping with these ethical issues).

## SUMMARY POINTS

- The challenges to governments worldwide to respond to the growing numbers of people with dementia are substantial. The response requires a public health approach to improve the care and experience of people with dementia and family caregivers. National approaches should be clearly articulated in either a stand-alone dementia policy or plan or by integrating a plan and policies within health, mental health or old-age policies.

- Some common factors are noted from the countries that have developed a policy or plan, namely:
  - The issues that need to be addressed broadly include raising awareness, timely diagnosis, commitment to good quality continuing care and services, caregiver support, workforce training prevention and research.
  - A sustainable financial commitment is crucial for the successful implementation of plans and programmes.

- Adequate financial and social support is essential for the protection of human rights for people with dementia and their caregivers and should be integrated into the policy or plan.

- Ethical principles that recognize fundamental human rights – including inclusivity and equitable access to resources and care, for all members of society regardless of social and cultural background and geographical location – should underpin policies, plans, legislation and practice guidelines.

- Education and support relating to ethical decision-making should be an essential part of capacity-building for all involved in providing dementia care, including policy-makers, professionals and families.

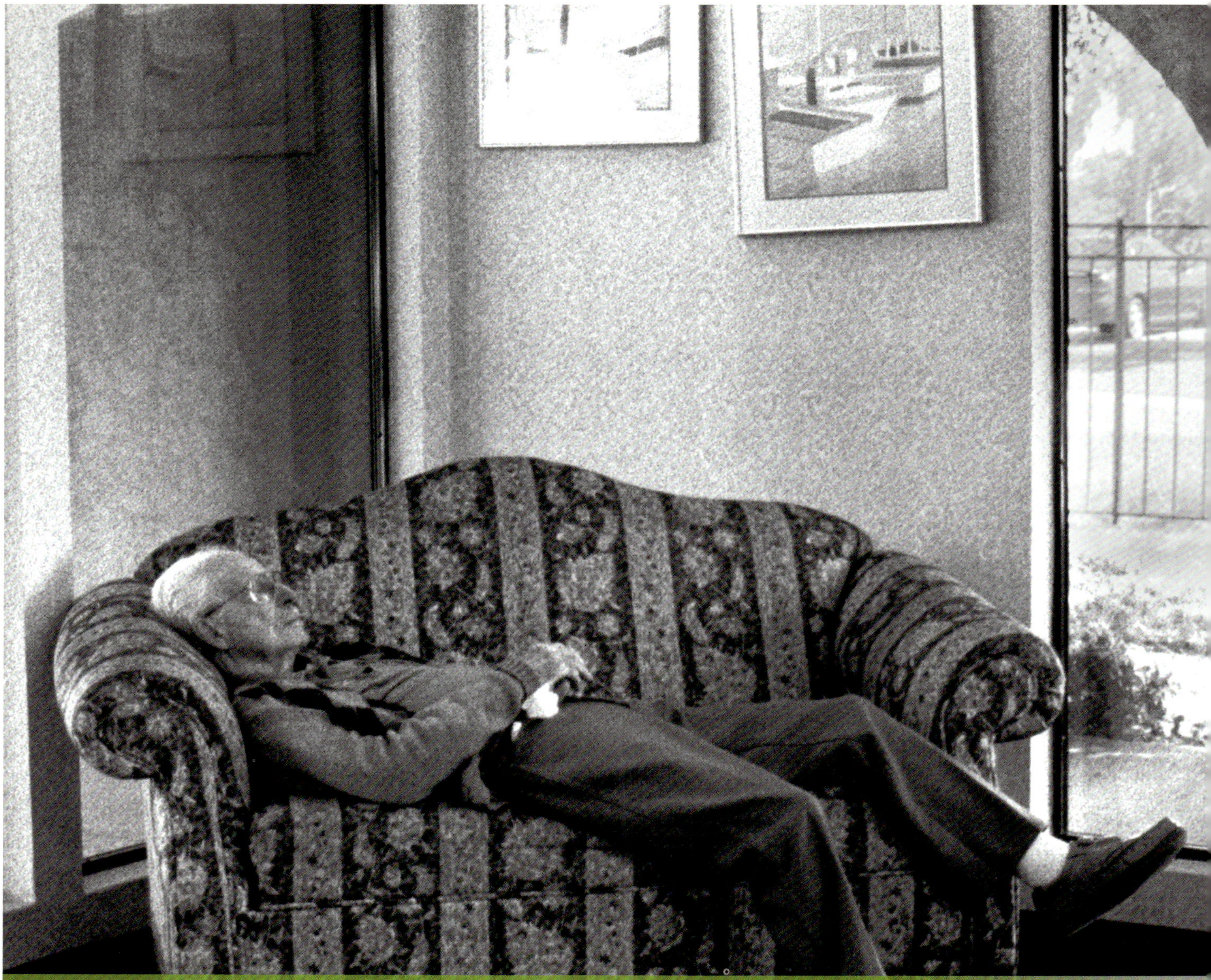

CHAPTER 4

# DEMENTIA HEALTH AND SOCIAL CARE SYSTEMS AND WORKFORCE

The demographic, economic and burden analyses of dementia challenge governments to develop and improve services for people with dementia, with an emphasis on earlier diagnosis, provision of support in the community, and a responsive health and social care sector. A few countries have recognized dementia as a priority, as described in chapter 3, by developing dementia policies, plans or strategies. However, these do not necessarily lead to action, and there appear to be barriers to the detection and management of dementia worldwide.

Health and social care systems must address both the substantial need for help from others that is required by people with dementia and the significant impact on caregivers. This chapter reviews the role of health and social support systems and their capacity to provide clinical management and long-term care for people with dementia. Strategies for enhancing receptivity and capacity within the workforce, such as the development of dementia care guidelines, are presented.

# HEALTH AND SOCIAL CARE SYSTEMS

## CARE PATHWAY FOR A PERSON WITH DEMENTIA

Dementia is associated with complex needs and, especially in the later stages, high levels of dependency and morbidity. These care needs, which include identification, diagnosis and symptom management as well as long-term support, often challenge the skills and capacity of the workforce and services. In addition, a substantial proportion of dementia care takes place outside formal health care settings and is provided by family members. To improve the quality of life of people with dementia and their caregivers, it is essential that the care provided by health and social care services is coordinated and integrated and can be adapted to the changes that occur throughout the course of the disease. A care pathway that is responsive to these changes and includes regular reassessment is key to improving the care of people with dementia.

### UNDERSTANDING THE DEMENTIA DIAGNOSTIC AND TREATMENT GAP

Dementia is under-diagnosed worldwide, and when a diagnosis is made it is typically at a relatively late stage in the disease process. Even in high-income countries only one fifth to one half of cases of dementia are routinely recognized and documented in primary care case note records *(179)*. There is only one such study conducted in a LMIC country (India) and, in this study, 90% of people with dementia had not received any diagnosis, treatment or care *(180)*. Both demand- and supply-side factors interact, highlighting the importance of understanding the links between health seeking behaviour, health and social service availability and a preparedness to understand the diagnostic and treatment gap.

A consultation exercise conducted for the *National Dementia Strategy* in England highlighted a combination of three factors contributing to low rates of detection of dementia – the stigma of dementia preventing open discussion, the false belief that memory problems are a normal part of ageing, and the false belief that nothing can be done. These factors resulted in inactivity in seeking and offering help *(121)*. Raising awareness and help-seeking are thus central to the strategy for reducing the dementia treatment gap. This will be discussed in greater detail in chapter 6.

Diagnosis of dementia requires effective coordination between primary and specialist care services. However, many of the health systems around the world are hampered by non-availability of adequately skilled providers. Figure 4.1 shows the difference in the number of psychiatrists per 100 000 population between countries *(147)*. Table 4.1 presents the difference in the number of a range of health professionals per 100 000 population according to World Bank income groups *(147)*. These results clearly show the limited number of human resources in the health sector in LMIC.

The roles of different cadres of health care providers in dementia care were examined on the basis of data collected through the WHO dementia survey. Neurologists and psychiatrists were most frequently identified with diagnosing and managing dementia. Primary care physicians, geriatricians and nurse practitioners were less likely to be involved in diagnosis. Survey respondents were asked to estimate the percentage of people likely to receive a diagnosis. The majority of respondents from LMIC (16 of 22; 45.4%) reported that fewer than 25% of people are diagnosed by one of the clinicians listed above. According to the survey respondents, memory or geriatric clinics exist for diagnosis, assessment and management in all participating high-income countries and in 16 of 22 (72.7%) of responding LMIC. However, 13 of the low-income countries reported that these facilities have limited geographical coverage and, in most cases, exist only n the capital city or in other large cities.

## ORGANIZING THE HEALTH CARE PATHWAYS

A dementia care pathway should be embedded in a health system that is resourced with trained providers who are able to make an accurate diagnosis in a timely and efficient manner, and that can link people to the provision of appropriate and adequate care as and when required. The important role of primary care has been neglected until recently. The extent and nature of the roles of the providers are dependent on the resource level of the health system.

The *World Alzheimer Report* 2009 provides a framework for planning dementia services *(3)*. It proposes a range of services reflecting the progressive nature of dementia and for planning collaboratively with community-based social care and support services (Figure 4.2). Governments in Australia, France and the United Kingdom are already working along these lines. Box 4.1 describes MAIA, a strategy adopted in the French Alzheimer Plan for a person-centred approach and to facilitate better coordination of different services.

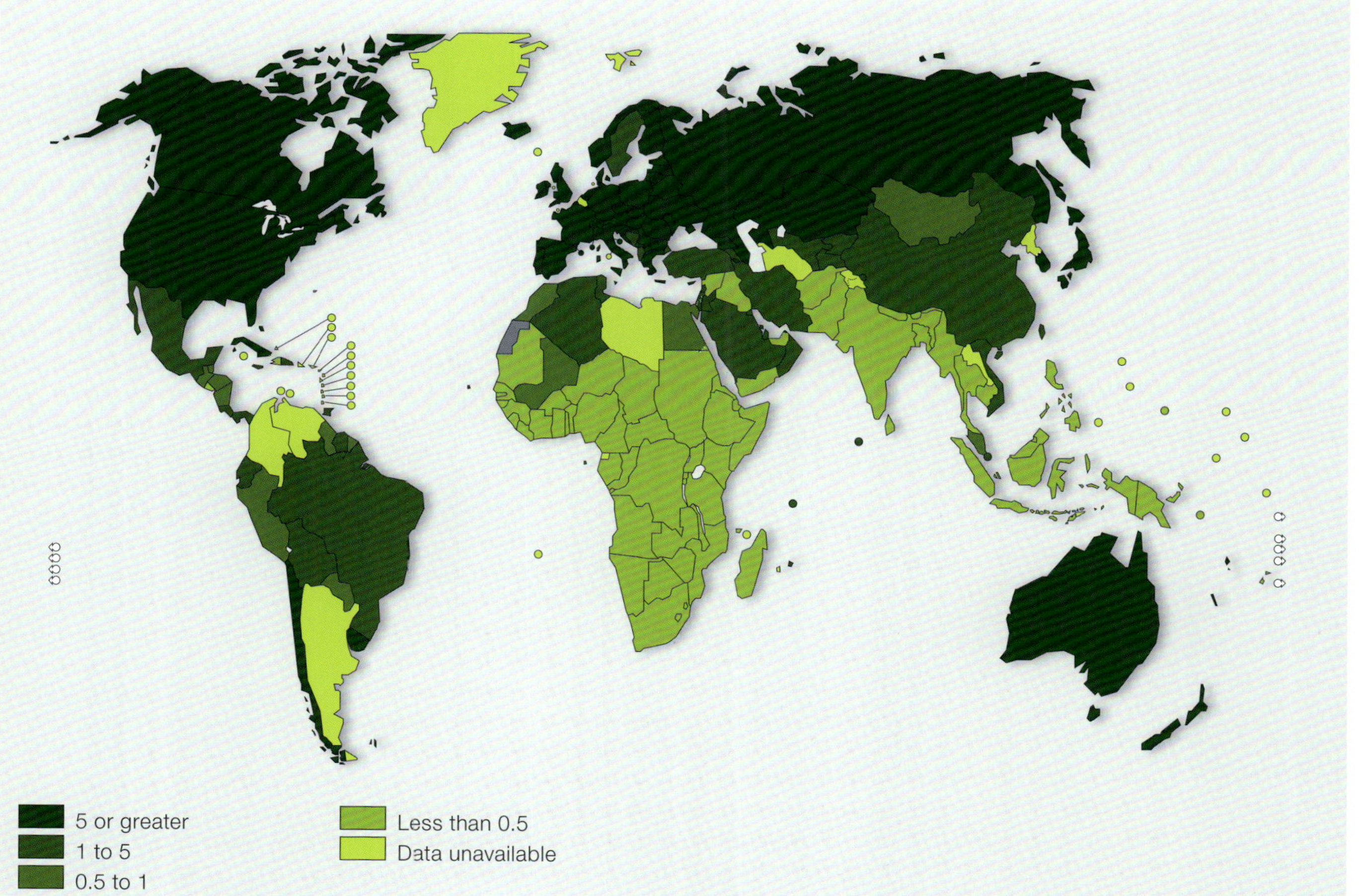


FIG. 4.1 Number of psychiatrists per 100000 population *(147)*

| Income Group | Psychiatrists | Other medical doctors | Nurses | Psychologists | Social workers | Occupational therapists | Other health workers |
|---|---|---|---|---|---|---|---|
| Low | 0.05 | 0.06 | 0.42 | 0.02 | 0.01 | 0.00 | 0.12 |
| Lower-Middle | 0.54 | 0.21 | 2.93 | 0.14 | 0.13 | 0.01 | 1.33 |
| Upper-Middle | 2.03 | 0.87 | 9.72 | 1.47 | 0.76 | 0.23 | 13.07 |
| High | 8.59 | 1.49 | 29.15 | 3.79 | 2.16 | 1.51 | 15.59 |
| **World** | **1.27** | **0.33** | **4.95** | **0.33** | **0.24** | **0.06** | **2.93** |

TABLE 4.1 Median rate of human resources per 100 000 population working in the mental health sector by World Bank income group *(147)*

BOX 4.1

## MAIA (MAISONS POUR L'AUTONOMIE ET INTÉGRATION DES MALADES ALZHEIMER) IN FRANCE

MAIAs are a key component of the French Alzheimer Plan aiming to provide better reception, orientation and care for persons with dementia. The MAIA model aims to reduce uncertainty for families who do not know who to contact and who would otherwise have to negotiate a maze of separate and poorly coordinated systems.

The MAIA solves this problem by creating a process of integration through a network of partners in the field of care, assistance and support in the local settings, such as hospitals, general practitioners, day care centres, Alzheimer's disease centres, council services, social services, home workers, volunteers, dementia associations etc. The goal is to offer a one-stop shop, irrespective of the organization through which the person first enters the system. The response must also be as comprehensive as possible. The MAIA system does not replace the existing system but provides the structure for improved coordination. The MAIA provides services in response to the needs expressed by the persons concerned, rather than the resources that happen to be in place.

Fifteen trials have demonstrated that MAIA works at subdepartment level. The trials show that local coordination is necessary to achieve a first level of integration and to allow case managers (for complex cases) to act effectively. Scaling up has begun and, by 2014, 500 MAIA will provide full coverage of France.

*Source: Reference 125.*

### THE ROLE OF PRIMARY CARE

It is widely accepted that the initial identification of likely cases of dementia is an important function of primary care. Many suggest that formal diagnosis should be done by specialists, as explicitly stated in France's Alzheimer Plan *(125)*, and is implicit in the United Kingdom's policy *(121)*, in that determining eligibility for, and initiation of, anti-dementia drug prescriptions should be carried out only by specialists in the field. Because primary care has an important role to play, it would be challenging to decrease the treatment gap even in well-resourced high-income countries without effective coordination between primary care and specialist services.

In LMIC, primary care and non-specialists have a much bigger role to play in diagnosing and managing dementia because of insufficient numbers of specialists (Figure 4.1). Furthermore, outreach in the community and regular home visits are important for identifying older persons with early-stage dementia. WHO has identified dementia as one of the priority conditions to be addressed in its Mental Health Gap Action Programme (mhGAP), particularly in LMIC *(181)*. Within this programme, evidence-based guidelines have been developed for the management of dementia by non-specialists with a view to scaling up treatment and reducing the treatment gap *(9)* (Box 4.2).

| Pre-diagnosis | Diagnosis | Post-diagnostic support | Co-ordination and care management | Community services | Continuing care | End of life palliative care |
|---|---|---|---|---|---|---|
| Public awareness of the disease, its symptoms and where to go for help if someone is worried that they may have dementia | Receiving the diagnosis | Information and support for the person with dementia and their family caregivers to enable them to come to terms with the disease, plan for the future and make the best use of their current circumstances; continuing to do what they can still do and not concentrating on declining abilities | Assessing (and regularly reassessing) the needs of people with dementia and arranging care in conjunction with them and their caregivers | This is when care is needed at increasingly short intervals, behavioural and psychological symptoms become more prevalent and the person with dementia is less able to care for themselves; care may be provided in the person with dementia's own home or community facilities | Care is needed continuously, unpredictable or behavioural and psychological symptoms become more demanding; this stage should also include when people with dementia require hospital care for whatever reason | This is the special form of continuing care when a person with dementia is close to the end of his or her life |

The co-ordination and care management stage should apply throughout the journey of dementia care from diagnosis to palliative care.

**FIG 4.2** Seven-stage model for planning dementia services *(3)*

## LONG-TERM CARE SERVICES

Effective coordination of ongoing health and social care services after diagnosis is vital for achieving improved quality of life for people with dementia and their caregivers beyond the pre-diagnostic and diagnostic phases which are health-system based. A wide variety of services for post-diagnostic support, community services, services for continuing care and end-of-life palliative care are also essential (Figure 4.2).

The term "long-term care" is often used to describe the range of services which help meet both the medical and nonmedical need of people with a chronic illness or disability who cannot care for themselves. Long-term care includes:

- *post-diagnostic services:* planning for the future; offering support, advice and information as needed; and helping maintain independence;
- *community services:* helping people with dementia to remain at home as long as they wish and until it is no longer possible, and providing short breaks/respite care to support caregivers and providing an opportunity for social engagement for the recipient.
- *continuing care:* caring for people who can no longer stay at home (e.g. in different kinds of supported or institutional living arrangements such as group homes and residential care), and providing for the end stages of dementia.

As the aims are interlinked, coordination is required across the range of services to provide a seamless response and a partnership approach. Long-term care can be both formal and unpaid/informal. Unpaid care is the care provided by family and friends. Formal care is care provided by paid caregivers and can include nursing care and personal care provided in a care home or domiciliary setting.

The majority of people with dementia live in their own homes in the community. Moreover, most people would wish to remain living in their own homes for as long as possible. This message is consistently given by the public, by older people generally, and by people with dementia specifically. In addition, economic research carried out in high-income countries has shown that the largest cost driver for dementia is the cost of institutional care *(3)*.

Most high-income countries are moving, or trying to move, away from the institutional traditions of the early part of the past century, not only for major mental disorders but also for the care of older adults (with health problems). States now prioritize community-based care systems. It is estimated there are 266 574 people with dementia in Australia in 2011. This is projected to increase to 553 285 people by 2030, and 942 624 people by 2050 *(182)*. In response, Commonwealth and State Australian governments have developed comprehensive plans and systems including expansion of community care services and packages, improvement in quality of residential care and initiatives to address behavioural and psychological symptoms of dementia *(183)*. Some countries, including Japan and Sweden, have introduced small group homes as an

BOX 4.2

## MENTAL HEALTH GAP ACTION PROGRAMME (MHGAP)

WHO developed the Mental Health Gap Action Programme (mhGAP) in 2008 with the objective of scaling up care for mental, neurological and substance use (MNS) conditions in LMIC. The mhGAP strategy supports an integrated approach for the management of priority MNS conditions, including dementia, within and outside the health sector. The goal of mhGAP is to close the GAP between what is urgently needed and what is currently available in order to reduce the burden of MNS conditions worldwide by:

- reinforcing the commitment of stakeholders to increase the allocation of financial and human resources;
- achieving higher coverage of key interventions, especially in LMIC.

The mhGAP intervention guide for MNS conditions in non-specialist health settings is a technical tool developed by WHO to assist in implementation of mhGAP. The intervention guide was developed through a systematic review of evidence followed by an international consultative and participatory process. The guide presents integrated management of priority conditions using protocols for clinical decision-making.

The intervention guide is a model that can be used by health care providers working in non-specialized health care settings, following adaptation for national and local needs.

*Source: References 9 and 181.*

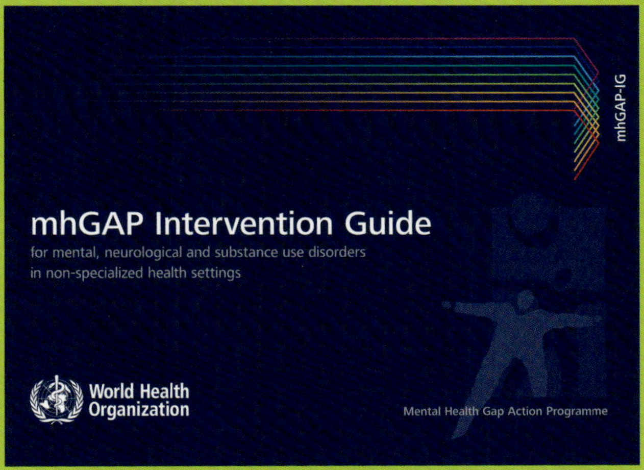


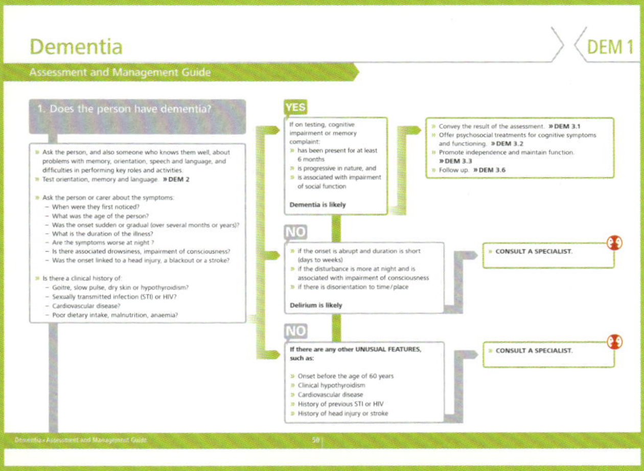


mhGAP intervention guide dementia algorithm

intermediate level of care between home and institutional care. Small group homes accommodate groups of 6–10 residents who are supported by staff around the clock. Group home living provides an alternative to traditional institutionalization / residential care when there is a lack of informal or formal community support *(184)*.

In LMIC in Africa, Asia and Latin America, formalized institutional care for the older people is rare. Long-term care remains a family responsibility to a great extent. Most families cannot afford private care and few state-funded facilities exist. The available institutional care tends to be provided by faith-based and other nonprofit organizations, as in Mexico (Box 4.3).

BOX 4.3

## DAY-CARE CENTRES FOR PEOPLE WITH DEMENTIA IN MEXICO

Mexico has a population of 112 million and almost 10% of them are over 60 years of age. Around 600 000 people are estimated to have dementia.

Mexico currently has no government programme to meet the needs of people with dementia and their caregivers. There are seven registered day-care centres for people with dementia in Mexico. All the centres are run by NGOs, mostly through initiatives of the Mexican Alzheimer associations. All are based in the large cities, including two in Mexico City. All have multidisciplinary well trained teams but only around 30 people can attend to each day-care centre. The existing centres are clearly insufficient to meet the needs of the population.

The day-care centres are financed primarily by donations and small payments from the users and their families. They are administered by a board of trustees. A more secure scheme of funding is necessary to scale up the number of these centres.

*Source: Reference 185.*

BOX 4.4

## A TWO-WEEK RESPITE PROGRAMME FOR CAREGIVERS AND PERSONS WITH DEMENTIA IN AUSTRIA

This programme provides care for both the caregiver and the person with dementia. Between 10 and 15 "pairs" (caregiver and person with dementia) join each programme. While people with dementia receive individual stage-specific stimulation (e.g. cognitive and memory training, occupational therapy, physical training), caregivers take part in an intensive training course in which they learn about the disease and are trained in special communication techniques. They receive group and individual counselling. Caregivers also have the freedom to use the time as they please, to relax and take time off.

The effectiveness of this programme with regard to perceived burden and depressive symptoms of caregivers was evaluated in a single group, pre-post-design assessing 104 caregivers. The results indicated that depressive symptoms and the burden related to symptoms of the disease were reduced during the treatment. The programme was well received and accepted by caregivers and patients. More than 30 such courses have been held so far since 2000.

*Source: References 188, 189.*

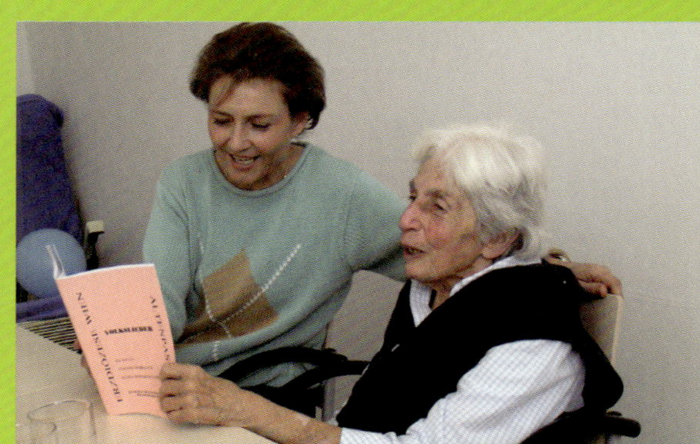

*Photo credit: M.A.S Alzheimerhilfe, Austria/Stefanie Auer*

### COMMUNITY SERVICES

The right support at the right time and in the right place is especially important for giving people with dementia both choice and control over the decisions that affect them. Support is required for people residing in the community for a wide range of services, including housekeeping, cooking, shopping, transport, and personal care assistance such as help with personal hygiene.

Six of seven (85.7%) WHO dementia survey respondents from high-income countries reported that community services are provided to people with dementia, compared with 3 of 21 (14.2%) respondents from LMIC. China and Russia, for example, reported that services are limited to major cities. All the countries providing community services indicated that care workers are involved in the provision of care. In some countries, including Canada, care workers are supervised by trained or licensed health professionals.

WHO dementia survey respondents from high-income countries reported that community services are provided under a range of funding options – full fee-paying, subsidized or free. In Japan, for instance, services are covered by long-term care insurance with co-payment (Box 3.6).

### RESPITE CARE

Most family caregivers wish to be able to provide support to help the person with dementia stay at home. However, providing care at home may place stress on the caregiver, leading to a range of adverse effects both on the caregiver and the recipient of care (see chapter 5). To provide adequate care at home, the caregiver may require assistance from formal services. Respite care is the temporary provision of care for a person with dementia by people other than the primary caregiver. The term "respite care" is used to cover a diverse range of services. Respite care can take place in the home of the person with dementia, in a day-care centre, in the community (e.g. attending a social event) or in a residential setting. It may vary in terms of who provides the care (trained or untrained staff or volunteers). Respite care may also vary in duration – ranging from a few hours to a several weeks – and may involve daytime-only care or overnight care. Respite care may be planned or, in an emergency, unplanned.

The aim of respite care is to give the primary caregiver respite from his or her caregiving responsibilities and hopefully ameliorate, to some degree, the stresses associated with being a caregiver. Respite services should also benefit the person with dementia. High-quality respite can provide opportunities for engagement and socializing *(186)* (Box 4.4). Evidence regarding the effectiveness of respite care is limited. A review of three randomized controlled trials showed no benefit on any outcome for caregivers *(187)*. However, a host of methodological problems in available trials were identified, indicating the need for further research in this area.

In the WHO dementia survey, 5 out of 8 (62.5%) high-income country respondents reported that the country provided respite services, compared with 3 out of 22 (13.6%) LMIC country respondents. However a further three respondents from LMIC reported that respite is available from a private provider or from the local Alzheimer organization. Furthermore, the cost of respite services is generally subsidized in high-income countries, whereas the full cost of respite is more likely to be borne by the recipient in LMIC.

### RESIDENTIAL CARE

Despite a shift in priority in high-income countries to community service provision, residential care is still a significant feature of long-term care for people with dementia, and it may be the most appropriate and effective way of meeting someone's needs and providing a service of choice when community support (formal and informal) is insufficient.

Seven out of eight (87.5%) survey respondents from high-income countries reported that their country provides support (via funding or resources) for residential care, compared with 8 out of 22 (36.4%) respondents from LMIC. Even when present, many a times the number of facilities is insufficient. For example, Poland reported there is just one facility designed for people with dementia in the country. All but one of the countries with government-supported residential care facilities reported that they are regulated by a government department. However, only three countries reported that the regulations were sufficient. The inadequacy in regulations is reportedly due to limited funding to enforce them, too few prosecutions of facilities occur that do not follow them, and too few regulations specific to dementia care. At the time of the survey, the Dominican Republic was developing regulations.

A recognition of the need to improve the standard and quality of residential care has seen the emergence of alternative models of care, some of which have influenced the philosophy and practice of care provision in facilities in some high-income countries. Among these, the work of Tom Kitwood *(190, 191)*, who coined the term "person-centred care", is well known. Kitwood was critical of what he termed "the old culture of care" which reduces dementia to a biomedical approach and ignores subjectivity (the lived experience). For Kitwood, the old culture of care is task-driven and focused on medical approaches to care. In contrast, person-centred care is value-driven and focuses on the well-being and empowerment of people with dementia and their families.

Other models, such as dementia care mapping, adopt the principles of person-centred care. Dementia care mapping is an assessment tool and philosophy designed to improve person-centred care. The findings of a clustered randomized controlled trial with 325 participants from residential care facilities in Australia compared outcomes for residents assigned to one of three groups: person-centred care, dementia care mapping, or traditional care. Residents assigned to dementia care mapping and person-centred care showed improvement in agitation compared with participants receiving normal care *(192)*.

### PALLIATIVE CARE

Palliative care has been defined by WHO as "an approach that improves the quality of life of patients and their families facing the problems associated with life-threatening illness, through the prevention and relief of suffering by means of early identification and impeccable assessment and treatment of pain and other problems, physical, psychosocial and spiritual" *(193)*. It should include support and bereavement counselling for families *(194)*.

Evidence exists that the care of people with dementia, especially towards the end of their lives, is less than optimal *(195)*. Palliative care stands well with the aims of person-centred dementia care and is beneficial in relation to caring for people with dementia. Palliative care, and particularly end-stage palliative care, should ideally be managed by clinicians or others who have knowledge and experience of the issues that are likely to occur (including pain, refusal of food and fluids, inability to swallow and, for the caregivers, bereavement and adjusting to a non-curative approach to treatment) *(196)*.

## ORGANIZING LONG-TERM CARE SERVICES

Both LMIC and high-income countries are faced with the increasing need for provision of long-term care for the ageing population generally, and for people with dementia more specifically.

High-income countries have seen rapid escalations in the cost of long-term care, whether provided by the state, by the private sector or by families *(197)*. The demand for long-term care services is set to rise sharply with the increase in the ageing population. This is generating intense debate about the funding and form of future provision. Currently, the scale, form and quality of long-term care provision in high-income countries is variable, suggesting that there is considerable scope for sharing and learning from different national experiences *(198, 199)*.

**BOX 4.5**

## CARE FOR PEOPLE WITH DEMENTIA IN MALAYSIA

In Malaysia, the Ministry of Health Social Welfare Department provides services for older adults, including health care, guidance, counselling, recreation, religious teaching and welfare services. Financial assistance and institutional care is provided to those without a family and to the indigenous population through social services. Persons aged 60 years and above who are registered with the Social Welfare Department are given a monthly allowance under the Aid for Older Persons scheme. These older adults are also entitled to a discount when purchasing artificial/orthopedic appliances and spectacles, and for domestic travel. The ministry also administers day-care centres for elderly persons who live in the community.

Many NGOs are involved in providing community services to older people. They include palliative home care provided by Hospis Malaysia and day-care centres. Day-care centres provide care for the elderly person while the caregiver goes to work. These care resources and systems also cater for older adults who may develop dementia.

*Source: Reference 200.*

Meeting the challenges of growing long-term care needs is fundamentally a matter of public choice and political will. This can be seen in OECD countries where differing priorities given to long-term care reflect wide variations in public and private spending (from 0.6% of GDP in Spain to 2.8% in Sweden) *(197)*. Differences in spending levels are mainly determined by how extensive the provision of state-provided services is and by the quality of care.

Supporting an older person in his or her own home generally costs less than accommodation in a nursing home or other residential care facility, and it is what most people want. However, to achieve this goal the country must ensure that a broad range of support services is available, including respite care and professional guidance to families *(197)*. The option of small group homes as an alternative to traditional nursing home forms of residential care should also be explored.

In many LMIC the belief persists that these needs can and are being met through family support, despite growing evidence to the contrary. In Malaysia the government has recognized the need for long-term care and is developing facilities both under government schemes and those run by NGOs (Box 4.5).

Responding to the challenge of long-term care requires difficult decisions and trade-offs regarding the role of state and society, the status of informal caregivers (who are predominantly women) and, in particular, the rights and entitlements of care recipients. Appropriate long-term care interventions can contribute to the function and the quality of life for people with dementia, reduce the need for expenditure on mainstream health services, and delay or reduce admission to residential care. It can also minimize the indirect costs to informal caregivers of reduced economic and social participation.

The challenge of organizing long-term care in developing countries requires strategies to ensure the efficient use of the scarce resources involving the primary and non-specialist service providers and also a focus on community outreach. Prince et al *(201)* propose a package of care for LMIC which extends the basic package and which focuses on diagnosis coupled with information, regular needs assessments, physical health checks, and caregiver support. This package should be extended to include caregiver training, respite care, and assessment and treatment of behavioural and psychological symptoms of dementia where possible. The authors also suggest that care can best be delivered by trained primary care teams, with a shift towards long-term care and community outreach. Equally, they observe that care delivery will be more efficient when integrated with that for other chronic diseases and with more broadly based community-support programmes for older people and for those living with disabilities.

Similarly, WHO's mhGAP *(9, 181)* approach which was discussed earlier focuses on the important role of non-specialist providers in diagnosing and managing cases of dementia and providing support to caregivers in the community. Within mhGAP and other such projects, there is need to generate evidence on the effectiveness of such strategies in inducing relevant and persistent system changes and in producing benefits at sustainable costs.

# CARE PATHWAYS FOR POPULATIONS WITH SPECIFIC NEEDS

Some groups have additional needs arising from having dementia or being a caregiver of a person with dementia. Examples of specific or minority groups include indigenous and ethnic minorities, migrants, people with intellectual disabilities, people who identify as gay, lesbian, bisexual, transsexual or transgender, and younger people with dementia.

Although each of these population groups has its own unique needs, there are certain commonalities. These groups are more likely to face difficulty in receiving a diagnosis, obtaining information about dementia and accessing health and social services than their mainstream counterparts. Some of the barriers to access include a lack of understanding or recognition of the dementia in their population group, language or cultural barriers, and a lack of appropriate information resources and services. For these reasons, policies and care pathways that are adapted to their particular needs, and that are delivered in ways that are accessible and acceptable, are necessary to enable these groups have equitable access to services.

The following examples demonstrate the ways in which flexibility in the translation of care pathways and policies can provide a broad reach of programmes and resources to all people in need of them.

### INDIGENOUS AND ETHNIC MINORITY GROUPS

In Australia, prevalence studies among remote dwelling Aboriginal and Torres Strait Islander (A&TSI) people have demonstrated a high risk for dementia *(202)*. Collaboration between A&TSI people and health and service providers has resulted in the identification of priorities for supporting A&TSI people with dementia, including early diagnosis and access to appropriate services, and at the same time maintaining cultural knowledge *(203)* (Box 4.6).

The diversity of ethnic minorities (including recent immigrants and those who are second- or third-generation migrants) brings its own set of challenges to responding to people with dementia and their families. Studies highlight how ethnic minority status negatively influences the use of services *(204, 205)*. In particular, understanding of dementia (including the belief that it is a normal part of ageing rather than a disease of the brain, and thinking there are spiritual explanations), experiences of shame or stigma from other members of their community, and past negative experiences with health

**BOX 4.6**

## DEMENTIA CARE IN ABORIGINAL AND TORRES STRAIT ISLANDER POPULATIONS IN AUSTRALIA

The Aboriginal and Torres Strait Islander (A&TSI) people of Australia face disadvantages regarding many health outcomes, including a lower life expectancy and, according to preliminary data, higher rates of dementia (4.8 times more likely than non-indigenous Australians). Social and health indicators, including poor diet, higher rates of chronic disease, trauma and lower education levels, also contribute to a higher risk of developing dementia.

Despite this, A&TSI peoples maintain their wisdom, knowledge and culture which is transferred orally across generations. This information includes bush medicines, socioemotional stories from families, land care, and bush foods.

A&TSI people, working in partnership with the national dementia organization, Alzheimer's Australia, have identified dementia care, services and support as a priority. Maintenance of cultural knowledge while improving access to modern health care will help to overcome some of the disadvantages A&TSI people currently face. Early diagnosis and local service provision from A&TSI people will help those with dementia to remain in their homes and local communities for as long as possible. Investment in long-term care, by improving the clinical skills of the A&TSI workforce, will also generate employment.

Enabling A&TSI people to care for A&TSI people with dementia, will also strengthen the social fabric for humane reasons. The willingness to provide care for someone helps in learning to be humble, patient and to share happiness. These humane qualities are important for maintaining functional interdependence and improving other social outcomes.

*Source: References 202, 208–210.*

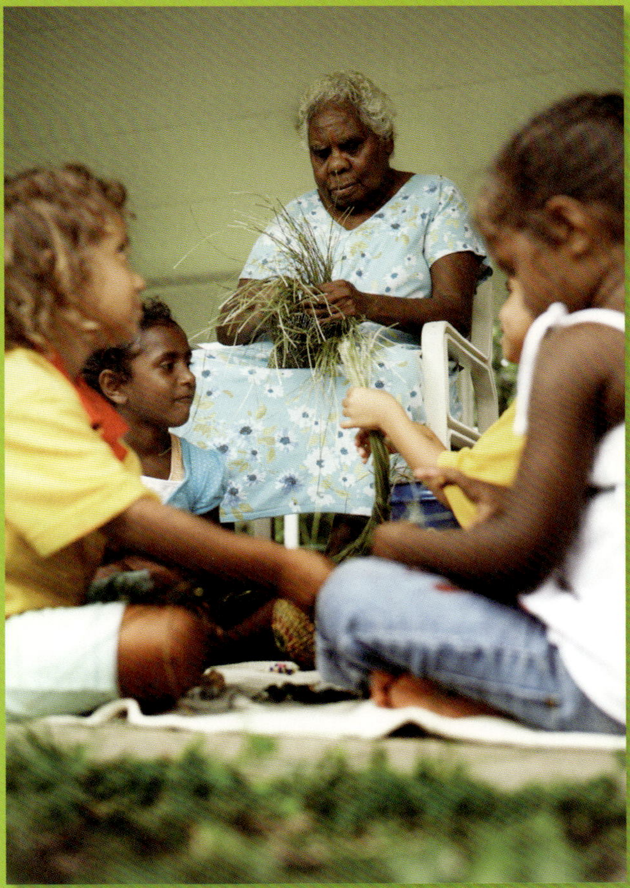

*Photo credit: Alzheimer's Australia Positive Images Series IV/ Lynton Crabb -Elder teaching children at Yarrabah Aged Person Hostel, Yarrabah Aboriginal Community*

**BOX 4.7**

## THE DEMENTIA CARE NETWORK IN THE NETHERLANDS

In the Netherlands, the government funded a programme to stimulate integrated care by building dementia care networks. This programme met several barriers, including lack of professional participation at the social level (for instance general practitioners). Despite the barriers, the participants observed major improvements in integrated care in dementia and moderate changes in working conditions. With the client-centred approach, 86% of the professionals reported improved familiarity with various informal caregivers' problems such as guilt and embarrassment about having coping difficulties. Of these professionals, 40% found that the programme helped them deal with these problems. Furthermore, 50% of the professionals reported improvement in their knowledge of options for referring clients. The participants, especially the nurses, noted that their collaborative dementia care competencies improved.

*Source: Reference 229.*

services, all create barriers to seeking help. While research has identified barriers to help seeking *(206, 207)*, further study is needed to fully understand the role that ethnicity and culture play in improving help-seeking. As with the example provided for A&TSI people, collaborative approaches that are responsive to cultural beliefs and needs are essential.

### GAY, LESBIAN, BISEXUAL AND TRANSSEXUAL AND TRANSGENDER PEOPLE

Policy issues for the gay, lesbian, bisexual and transsexual and transgender communities largely fall into the realm of rights of partners to take responsibility for the care and welfare of an affected partner, including substitute decision-making in health care and financial issues.

Depending on the local culture, Alzheimer societies in some countries provide targeted support and education programmes for these populations, usually in partnership with their community-based organizations. Online support groups are one way of reaching these communities who, for historical reasons of discrimination, may prefer to remain anonymous. Online support also provides flexibility for geographically dispersed groups, just as it does for any population group.

### INTELLECTUAL DISABILITY

People with Down syndrome are at a significant risk of developing Alzheimer's disease. Studies suggest that 50–70% will be affected by dementia after the age of 60 years. The onset of dementia in people with Down syndrome is likely to be younger than the sporadic form of dementia that generally affects older people *(211)*.

In the USA a national task force of experts on intellectual disabilities and Alzheimer's disease has developed a comprehensive report with policy and practice recommendations on detection, care and support for this population. The aim of the report is to enable adults with intellectual disabilities who are affected by dementia to remain living in the community with quality support *(211)*.

### PEOPLE WITH YOUNG ONSET DEMENTIA

The epidemiology of people with YOD (also referred to as early onset dementia in some of the literature) has been discussed in Chapter 2. From a social perspective, a person who develops dementia before nominal retirement age is differently placed in the lifespan compared with a person who develops dementia when older. Persons with YOD may still be working or may have recently left the workforce, they may have children still in the home or of university age, and they may not have the additional chronic conditions that the older population generally acquires. Furthermore, the information and support that is available to the older person with dementia is usually inappropriate.

From a policy perspective, the young onset population requires specific consideration because eligibility for social/medical supports or old age pensions is frequently based on an attained age, and younger persons may not be able to access financial support. People with YOD and those in the early stage of dementia are often engaged by dementia advocacy groups as spokespersons and advocates, and they frequently play a role in the governance of their organizations. This inclusion has led to positive policy recommendations in recognition of this niche population. To the extent that they engage in public activities and share their experiences, these younger faces of dementia can also provide a positive dissonance that helps mitigate the ageism that is associated with dementia.

## WORKFORCE CAPACITY-BUILDING

In this report, the health and social workforce is broadly defined as all people engaged in actions whose primary intent is to enhance health and well-being. This means that unpaid caregivers are in the workforce. However, for the purpose of this section we refer only to service providers in the health and social care sector. Unpaid caregivers are discussed in Chapter 5.

Within the health and social care sector many workers will assist people with dementia to varying degrees. Examples include: primary and community care (general practitioners, practice nurses, social workers, care coordinators, allied health professionals, personal assistants, domiciliary care, general and community hospitals), clinical and ancillary staff (including those providing clinical support), and staff in mental health services, rehabilitation services, care homes and palliative care services. Some of these workers provide long-term care in the community, including both health and social care.

## WORKFORCE ATTITUDES AND KNOWLEDGE

The attitudes of health and social care workers towards dementia are coloured by their experience, professional knowledge and skills, which in turn relate to the discipline and its position in the health care system. For instance, in several countries general practitioners are the gatekeepers to the health care system. Their decision on whether to pursue a diagnosis of dementia is crucial *(212)*. Yet early diagnosis does not occur often. One possible contributing factor is a knowledge gap *(213–216)*. General practitioners have highlighted their lack of knowledge about community services and resources, about making the diagnosis and the ability to distinguish between dementia and normal ageing (and the subsequent fear of making a false diagnosis), and about how to communicate the diagnosis *(216)*. Other themes which have been identified as potential barriers to diagnosis include perceived lack of available support services, therapeutic nihilism, late presentation (which is sometimes due to mistaking the signs of dementia for normal ageing), practitioners' own emotional responses and stigma *(216–218)*.

Some recent studies have specifically highlighted stigma as a factor that may interfere with timely diagnosis *(218–221)* and with communicating the diagnosis *(175, 218, 222, 223)*. On the basis of a five-country qualitative study involving multidisciplinary focus groups, the researchers concluded that stigma is the most powerful obstacle to timely diagnosis *(220)*. Stigma in relation to dementia is discussed more broadly in Chapter 6.

There is growing evidence that, even among those working in specialist dementia services, the proportion of staff receiving dementia care training is low *(224)*. For example, in the United Kingdom around one third of care homes with dedicated dementia provision report having no specific dementia training for staff *(144)* and 52% of nursing staff in hospitals *(225)* have not received any work-based professional development or learning opportunities in dementia care. Evidence also suggests a variable picture of the quality of current provision of dementia training *(224, 226)*.

## CAPACITY-BUILDING: KEY ISSUES

The following factors are important when examining the issue of capacity-building for the dementia workforce:

- the different stages of dementia and the different inputs needed at each stage;
- the competencies required to deliver high quality and safe services;
- numbers of different categories of the health and social workforce;
- the existing skills of different categories of service providers;
- the existence of continuing professional development and supervision to ensure regular assessment and support of competencies.

Based on above factors, a number of themes emerge that should be considered for capacity-building of the workforce.

### COMPETENCIES REQUIRED

Five core competencies have been identified for people requiring long-term care: person-centred care, partnering, quality improvement, information and communication technology, and a public health perspective *(227)*. The challenge is to translate these core competencies into practice through the institutions that produce and deploy the health workforce. Changes in the curriculum, new teaching methods and innovative training models are necessary. The case example from the Netherlands in Box 4.7 demonstrates movement in this direction.

### TRAINING NEEDS

There is a need for training in the basic medical, nursing and therapy curricula regarding diagnostic and needs-based assessments, and to move beyond the current preoccupation with simple curative interventions to encompass long-term support and chronic disease management. Given the frailty of many older people with chronic health conditions, there is also a need for training in outreach care, and in assessing and managing patients in their own homes.

### COLLABORATION AND TEAMWORK

Inherent in the new paradigm of care is a strong emphasis on collaboration and teamwork between different categories of health care provider and people with dementia and their families. Creating a relationship that values the role of the person with dementia and of the family as a partner in care has been frequently shown to improve health outcomes *(228)*. The multidisciplinary team includes psychiatrists, neurologists, psychologists, nurses, general practitioners, occupational therapists and community/social workers who can share their expertise and collaborate with each other The case example from India demonstrates a movement in this direction in Box 4.8.

BOX 4.8

## A MULTIDISCIPLINARY APPROACH TO ASSESSMENT AND MANAGEMENT IN INDIA

The assessment and management of dementia requires many different types of expertise and sometimes coordination is lost and the services are fragmented. To overcome this, the TS Srinivasan Institute, VHS Hospital, Chennai, India, established a multidisciplinary team. The team comprises a neurologist, psychiatrist, medical officers, clinical psychologists, counsellors, physical therapists, occupational therapists, and an electrophysiology technician. The team offers assessment and rehabilitation services for people with neurological and psychiatric disorders, including dementia.

After triage by the clinician, the patient with suspected cognitive impairment undergoes a detailed evaluation for psychosocial disability, physical disability and medical comorbidity. Laboratory tests and imaging are also carried out. The physician reviews the patient in light of the reports, concludes an assessment and offers treatment. If an individual is diagnosed as having early though established cognitive impairment, he or she is offered rehabilitation services such as physical and occupational therapy, with psychosocial interventions for the person and caregiver (including advocacy, cognitive retraining, nutritional counselling and wellness-enhancing treatments).

In this setting, the social worker or the nurse practitioner acts as the case manager. Establishing a firm link with the person with dementia and his/her family, the case manager provides and/or facilitates access to available services, acting as the liaison agent and optimizing the care and support services.

This multidisciplinary model of teamwork has considerable potential in the setting of LMIC as it reduces dependence on the doctor and allows scarce medical skills resources to be used optimally. It is also a model that has great acceptability, providing care beyond cure.

*Source: Reference 230.*

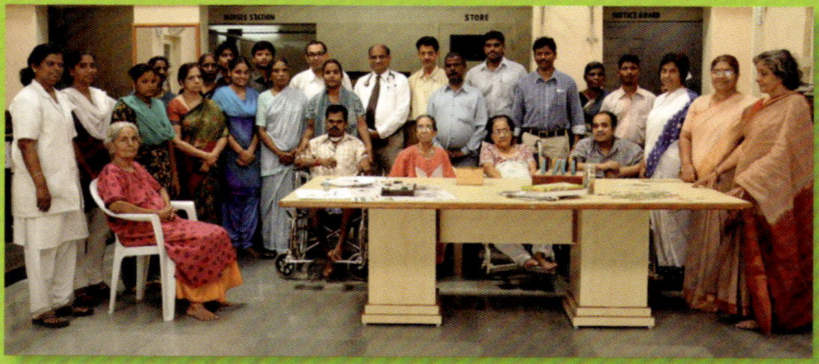

*Photo credit: The TS Srinivasan Institute, VHS Hospital, Chennai, India*

## LONG-TERM CARE WORKFORCE TRAINING: SPECIFIC ASPECTS

The long-term care workforce includes community nurses, health workers and residential care staff (including direct care workers). Non-professional direct care workers can help meet some of the demand for care as long as they are competent and supervised, and can draw upon professional staff when necessary to deal with complex cases.

In recent years there has been recognition of the need for special training for long-term care staff to enable them to respond appropriately to the needs of persons with dementia. Currently, efforts are being made to change educational curricula for nursing home staff and to establish psychosocial methodologies to improve care in nursing homes for people with dementia *(231, 232)*. For instance, special education in geriatrics and gerontology are offered in some countries. There are also examples from LMIC of training of the long-term care workforce in order to support dementia care in community. Kerala is a state located in south-west India. With highest life expectancy in India (74 years) and with a low rate of fertility, Kerala is undergoing demographic transition. In addition, a significant number of people have migrated to other countries, especially the Persian Gulf countries. Kerala therefore has a great need for support for care-dependent older people, and there are many agencies in the state that recruit women for home and institutional care. The Alzheimer's and Related Disorders Society of India has been conducting a Geriatric Care Training Programme (3–10 month duration) since 1993 in Kerala and other states *(233)*.

Dementia care training is especially needed for care workers who are responsible for the day-to-day physical care of this often highly care-dependent population. For example, in most states in Australia competency-based dementia training is a prerequisite for care workers in community-based and residential care *(183)*. In other countries the implementation of training of direct care staff has led to improved quality of care by reducing the frequency of interactional restraints and the severity of agitation *(234)*.

The scarcity of the health workforce in LMIC presents a special challenge *(227)*. An innovative strategy to overcome this scarcity is task shifting. The 10/66 dementia research group has tested the effectiveness of training community health care workers to deliver a brief intervention involving training of caregivers and this has been found to decrease caregivers' psychological morbidity and strain (Box 4.9).

## GUIDELINES FOR DEMENTIA CARE

The evidence to support practice guidelines in dementia care is more limited than in many other clinical areas, in part because of ethical concerns related to including people with dementia in research. However, this evidence is gradually growing.

Guidelines for dementia have been developed in a number of countries in recent years *(140, 238–240)*. Guidelines have also been developed by the Singapore Ministry of Health *(241)*. In addition, some countries have regional-level guidelines (as in Italy) *(241)*. From countries in Latin America, Argentina and Mexico have guidelines for dementia *(242–244)*. In addition, many professional associations have developed guidelines for dementia *(241)*. However, the guidelines differ in scope depending on the country-specific context and methodology. Guidance on the long-term care management of people with dementia is also of benefit to the workforce. An example of guidelines for long-term care in Australia is the Quality dementia care series *(245)*.

An important step for improving dementia care and services in LMIC has been the development of evidence-based guidelines by WHO *(246, 247)* in the area of dementia in its mhGAP programme. These form the basis of the WHO's mhGAP intervention guide for mental, neurological and substance use disorders for non-specialized settings *(9)*. The intervention guide contains simple clinical algorithms for primary care providers such as doctors and nurses (Box 4.2).

### GUIDELINES FOR DEMENTIA CARE: KEY ASPECTS

Guidelines for dementia care should include guidance on clinical aspects such as diagnosis, assessment and treatment, as well as quality long-term care. They should also include guidance on any legal and ethical issues that could compromise quality care.

The dementia strategy from England, *Living well with dementia: a national dementia strategy,* has outlined eight core principles for supporting people with dementia (Box 4.10). These are the areas for which guidance is required to enable the workforce to adequately support people with dementia and their caregivers. National guidelines should also be flexible enough to accommodate differences in regions and in cultural groups and, where required, should be translated into different languages and dialects.

**BOX 4.9**

## THE 10/66 DEMENTIA RESEARCH GROUP'S POPULATION-BASED "HELPING CARERS TO CARE" INTERVENTION

The 10/66 "Helping carers to care" train-the-trainer intervention was developed in India with input from the wider 10/66 group of international experts. It targets the main caregiver of the person with dementia and also includes members of the extended family. The aim is to provide the caregiver with basic education about dementia and specific training on managing behaviours that are problematic.

First, the community health workers are trained in a two-day training programme. They cover information provided in three modules and take part in role plays of intervention scenarios. The modules in the training package include:

**Module 1.** Assessment: a) Cognitive/functional impairment. b) Caregiver's knowledge and understanding of dementia. c) Care arrangements (Who are the family members? Who lives with the person with dementia? How do they assist the main caregiver? Which behavioural problems present most difficulties? How burdened do they feel?).

**Module 2.** Basic education: a) General introduction to the illness. b) What to expect in the future c) What causes/does not cause dementia? d) Locally-available care and treatment.

**Module 3.** Training on problem behaviours: Problem behaviours identified in the assessment are addressed (personal hygiene, dressing, incontinence, repeated questioning, clinging, aggression, wandering, apathy).

Second, the community health worker provides training to family caregivers over five weekly half-hour sessions.

The intervention has been tested in randomized controlled trials in Argentina, Chile, China, Dominican Republic, India, Mexico, Peru, Russia and Venezuela. The results indicated much larger treatment effects on caregiver psychological morbidity and strain than are typically seen in trials of such interventions in high-income countries.

*Source: References 235–237.*

### Clinical guidance

Depending on the context, clinical guidelines should:

- cover the broad scope of practice relating to the medical management of dementia, including diagnosis, assessment and management of symptoms;
- outline the benefits of early and accurate diagnosis for the person and family;
- provide a process of referral for specialist assessment and diagnosis where applicable (e.g. to a memory clinic or specialist physician);
- outline the criteria for pharmacological interventions, specifically the use of cholinesterase inhibitors;
- provide accurate information on behavioural and psychological symptoms of dementia;
- recommend nonpharmacological interventions as a first-line response to the behavioural and psychological symptoms of dementia;
- articulate the limitations and the risks associated with the use of antipsychotic medications as a response to behavioural and psychological symptoms of dementia (Box 4.11).
- include a caregiver assessment for burden and support needs.

### LONG-TERM CARE GUIDANCE

Comprehensive guidelines for long-term care for people with dementia will include the likely range of environments in which a person with dementia lives or is temporarily accommodated. These include the community, respite care and, when necessary, residential care. Other places where people may reside temporarily during the course of the disease include psychiatric or specialist units of care for those requiring assessment and management of complex behaviour and acute general hospitals.

Guidelines should provide clear steps for supporting physical and mental functioning and well-being for as long as possible. They should include guidance on the provision of:

- social engagement and recreational activities;
- cognitive stimulation and rehabilitation, where appropriate;
- physiological support, including identification and management of comorbid symptoms such as pain and delirium;
- environments that are both safe and stimulating;
- recognition of behavioural and psychological change and potential causes;

BOX 4.10

## EIGHT COMMON CORE PRINCIPLES FOR SUPPORTING PEOPLE WITH DEMENTIA

The following eight principles were developed for the Department of Health for England by working with employers, people with dementia, caregivers and provider organizations. They can be used to enable workforce development for any member of staff working in health or social care services with people at any stage of dementia, from the earliest signs to the fully diagnosed condition. The eight core principles are designed to be relevant to every setting and provide a basis for a general understanding of the condition. They aim to build workers' confidence in adapting their actions and communication in order to respond appropriately to the person with dementia.

**Principle 1:** Know the early signs of dementia.

**Principle 2:** Early diagnosis of dementia helps people receive information, support and treatment at the earliest possible stage.

**Principle 3:** Communicate sensitively to support meaningful interaction.

**Principle 4:** Promote independence and encourage activity.

**Principle 5:** Recognize the signs of distress resulting from confusion and respond by diffusing a person's anxiety and supporting their understanding of the events they experience.

**Principle 6:** Family members and other caregivers are valued, respected and supported just like those they care for and are helped to gain access to dementia care advice.

**Principle 7:** Managers need to take responsibility to ensure members of their team are trained and well supported to meet the needs of people with dementia.

**Principle 8:** Work as part of a multi-agency team to support the person with dementia.

*Source: Reference 248.*

**BOX 4.11**

## ISSUES IN THE USE OF ANTIPSYCHOTIC MEDICATION FOR PEOPLE WITH DEMENTIA

There has been increasing concern about the use of antipsychotic drugs for the management of behavioural and psychological symptoms in dementia. These drugs appear to be used too often and, at their likely level of use, potential benefits risks may be more than the benefits. This is a problem across the world.

Although the first-line treatment for behavioural and psychological symptoms of dementia is nonpharmacological, the prescription of psychotropic medication remains high and it appears that current systems deliver a largely antipsychotic-based response.

These drugs appear to have only a limited positive effect in treating these symptoms but can cause significant harm to people with dementia. The risks include cerebrovascular adverse events and mortality. Clearly, some people benefit from these medications (e.g. where there is severe and complex risk). However, the current level of use of antipsychotics for people with dementia presents a significant issue in terms of quality of care, with negative impacts in patient safety, clinical effectiveness and the patient experience.

The mounting body of evidence documenting these risks has led North American and European regulatory authorities to issue warnings against the use of atypical antipsychotics to treat patients with dementia, and the US Food and Drug Administration now requires both atypical and typical antipsychotic drugs to carry a "black box" warning label highlighting the increased risk of mortality. Despite these warnings, antipsychotic drug use still seems to be widespread, particularly in care settings. Studies indicate that prescribing rates for antipsychotic medication use in dementia varies from 20% to 33% and most cases are residing in nursing homes. Less is known of the use of these medicines in the community and in acute hospital settings.

Evidence exists that, in many cases, difficult behaviour can be safely managed by use of psychosocial interventions or a person-centred care approach. Staff should receive training and guidance in delivering psychosocial interventions. Antipsychotics should be considered as an option only in cases of imminent risk of harm to self and other. If these drugs must be used, they should be prescribed in low doses over short periods and maintained only if benefits are apparent. Discontinuation should be attempted regularly.

*Sources: References 249–253.*

- least restrictive management of behavioural and psychological symptoms (e.g. nonpharmacological approaches), including monitoring the effectiveness of the management approach;
- palliative support which is timely and ethically based;
- psychosocial support for the family.

Guidelines should acknowledge the importance of the relationship between the person with dementia, the family and the workforce (professionals and care workers), and should include guidance on processes for involving of each of these stakeholder in care planning with clearly defined boundaries.

Finally, guidelines should provide links to other related and supporting documents, including legal and regulatory guides and national or regional policies or plans.

## THE CHANGING DEMOGRAPHIC OF CARE WORKERS - THE MIGRANT WORKFORCE

Decisions surrounding training and recruitment must also take into account the distribution and type of workers required to meet the care needs of the population. An ageing population and a decrease in the availability of informal (family) caregivers have contributed to an increased demand for long-term care services in high-income countries *(254)*. This increase in demand requires an increase in the workforce which, in many countries, is being met by migrant health professionals and migrant care workers *(255, 256)*. In general, migration is from LMIC to high-income countries as people seek better working conditions (pull factors) *(227)*. Migrant workers (with a range of nationalities and from a variety of cultures) may have been influenced by factors shaping migration flows in the host country – including migration policies, humanitarian programmes, and recognition of qualifications *(255)* – or by push factors in the country of origin – such as poor living conditions or political unrest *(227)*. They may also differ as to whether they were recruited in their own country or on arrival to the host country. For instance, immigration may be contingent on securing employment first. In some LMIC, including China, rural-to-urban migration is meeting the increasing need for community support services.

Migrant care workers may face a number of challenges in the workplace, including language and communication barriers and cultural differences. Effective communication is particularly important when caring for people with dementia who, in many cases, will require assistance with communication themselves. Effective communication is also essential for liaising with family members and fellow staff members. Cultural differences may include lack of knowledge of local customs, laws and regulations; significant past events; and preferences regarding food preparation. Migrant care workers are vulnerable to abuse and exploitation such as inequity in pay and employment conditions and may experience discrimination and prejudice from co-workers, families and residents.

Measures that could improve the security of migrant care workers and which would result in the provision of better care outcomes for people with dementia and their families include the following:

- There should be an agreed definition of the term "migrant care worker" and established national data systems to identify numbers.

- A better understanding is required of migrant care workers' experience in the long-term care sector and, in particular, their experience of caring for people with dementia.

- Appropriate education and training should be provided, including with regard to language and culture. An example is the ASPIRE project in Scotland, which is run jointly by Alzheimer Scotland and local language tutors and which provides training for migrant workers in care homes. The aim of the training is to increase staff understanding of dementia and to improve communication with residents *(257)*.

- Appropriate human resource and regulatory support and protection need to be in place to prevent, and effectively manage, instances of exploitation, discrimination and abuse. The demand to balance the rights of migrant health workers with equity concerns related to an adequate health workforce in source countries has led to the development of ethical international recruitment policies, codes of practice and guidelines in some countries *(227)*.

## SUMMARY POINTS

- Countries should develop integrated and coordinated health and social pathways and services to cater for the changing needs of people with dementia and their caregivers. Such pathways and services should be inclusive of, and undertaken in collaboration with, specific population groups in order to ensure that their unique needs are identified and addressed.

- Greater community support, including respite options, will assist families to care for people with dementia for longer in community and will delay or reduce reliance on high-cost residential care.

- In resource-poor settings, a focus on community outreach could be an efficient use of scarce resources to improve the quality of life of people with dementia and their caregivers.

- Capacity-building in the workforce will contribute to improved integration and coordination of services. Multidisciplinary and coordinated action is required at all levels of the workforce.

- Workforce training curricula and programmes should be expanded to include education on dementia and management of long-term care and chronic diseases. The capacity of the health and social care workforce should be strengthened by developing appropriate guidelines in dementia care for both clinical and long-term care.

- The effectiveness of task-shifting (with appropriate guidelines and training) in LMIC should be further evaluated as a potential solution to the under-supply of a professional workforce.

- The growing migrant workforce in high-income countries has its own set of challenges that need to be understood and addressed.

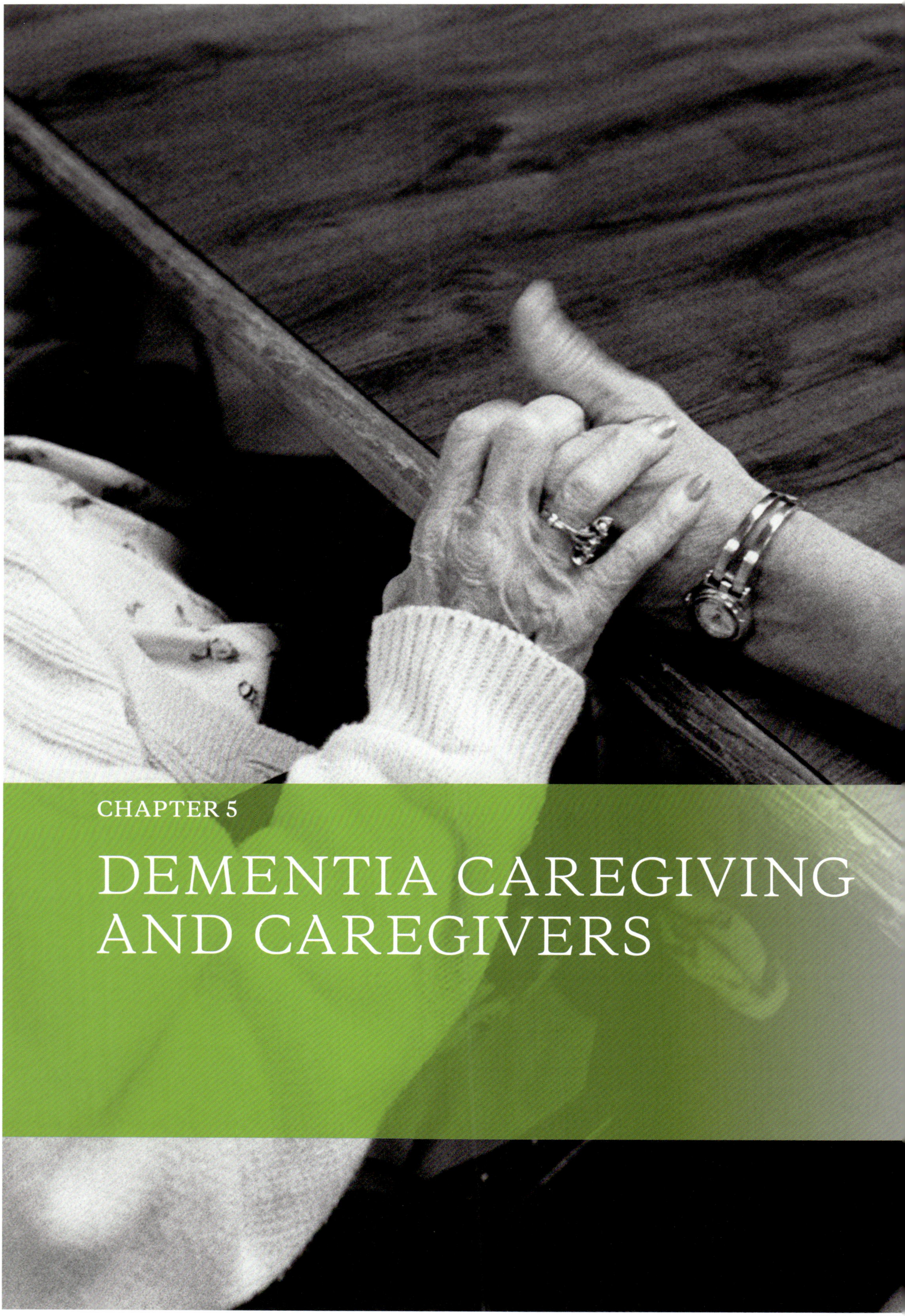

CHAPTER 5

# DEMENTIA CAREGIVING AND CAREGIVERS

Among chronic disease conditions, dementia has a uniquely profound effect upon disability and needs for care *(114, 258)*. Hence, it is important to consider the impact of the condition not only on the persons affected but also on their families, co-residents, neighbours and others in their networks – most particularly the persons who take the primary role in providing care.

All over the world, the family remains the cornerstone of care for older people who have lost the capacity for independent living. In high-income countries, the vital caring role of families, and their need for support, is often overlooked. In LMIC the reliability and universality of the family care system is often overestimated.

Shultz (2004) defines the role of caregiving as:

"... the provision of extraordinary care, exceeding the bounds of what is normative or usual in family relationships. Caregiving typically involves a significant expenditure of time, energy, and money over potentially long periods of time; it involves tasks that may be unpleasant and uncomfortable and are psychologically stressful and physically exhausting" *(259)*.

Most research into caregiving in dementia is cross-sectional, capturing snapshots in time. However, for caregivers and care recipients it is a long-term evolving process with key transition phases, sometimes referred to as the caregiving "career". The onset of caring is often hard to define; it tends to emerge naturally from customary family transactions, involving support given and received, that existed before the onset of dementia. The need for care may precede or post-date a formal diagnosis of dementia. Needs for care tend to escalate over time, from increased support for household, financial and social activities, to personal care, and to what for some is almost constant supervision and surveillance. Important transitions include the involvement of professional caregivers, institutionalization and bereavement.

In this chapter and throughout this report the term "caregiver" is used to describe those who provide informal unpaid care. "Carer" and "care provider" are synonymous terms or descriptions often used in literature. Informal caregivers can be taken to include all family members, friends, neighbours and other unpaid individuals providing regular care and / or supervision. People with dementia who need care are described as "care recipients".

This chapter begins with a demographic profile of those who care including, what they do and why. The impact of caregiving on family members, and particularly the primary caregiver, is discussed and there is an overview of intervention models that have been shown to reduce the stress associated with caregiving. The chapter also discusses barriers to service access and uptake and offers suggestions for improving support to caregivers in different contexts.

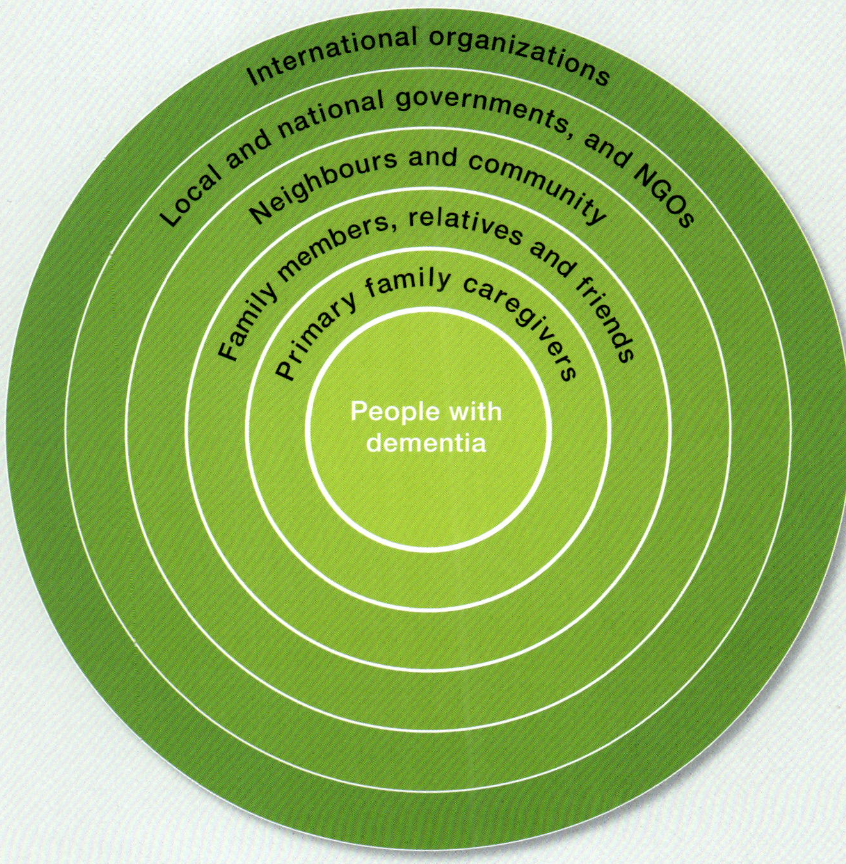
International organizations
Local and national governments, and NGOs
Neighbours and community
Family members, relatives and friends
Primary family caregivers
People with dementia

**FIG 5.1** The integrated caregiving system

## WHO CARES?

Caregiving and support is not the responsibility solely of the family and others in the immediate network of the person with dementia. It should also be a concern for communities, governments and society as a whole, although lack of awareness or commitment may mean that this is not the case in practice. Figure 5.1 illustrates levels of care (some very direct, such as that of family and neighbours; others less direct, but nevertheless crucial, such as the supportive role of government and society) and their proximity to the person at the centre of the arrangements for care, i.e. the person with dementia. The key role of family caregivers is often neither supported nor properly acknowledged.

Family caregivers can be defined by the relationship (spouse, adult children, daughters- and sons-in-law, friends, neighbours), primacy (primary or secondary caregiver), living arrangements (co-resident with the care recipient or living separately) and care input (regular, occasional or routine). Family caregivers can be involved in providing "hands-on" care or – also a very significant role – in organizing care delivered by others, sometimes from a distance. Primary caregivers are "persons, who spent most of the time with the person with dementia", and secondary caregivers, are those family and friends who "play a supplementary role to the care of a relative" *(260)*.

In most settings, most caregivers are spouses, and women outnumber men *(261–264)*. In the 10/66 Dementia Research Group population-based study in 11 sites in Latin America, China and India, women predominated as caregivers, except in rural China (Table 5.1). The Europe-based EUROFAMCARE study *(265)* of all caregivers of older people (not only caregivers of people with dementia) indicated that 76% are women (primarily wives, daughters and daughters-in-law). Similarly in Australia, women comprise 71% of co-resident primary caregivers *(266)*.

In the EUROCARE study which included 280 spouse caregivers from 14 European countries, in most countries (excluding Greece, Italy and Spain) the norm was for the married couple to be living on their own *(267)*. A multicentre pilot study including 706 caregivers of people with dementia in Latin America, India and China *(268)* found living alone or with a spouse was uncommon, this finding being confirmed in the population-based phase of the project *(3)* (Table 5.1). Indeed, in most

BOX 5.1

## CARE FOR OLDER ADULTS IN NIGERIA

In Nigeria, the extended family kinship system persists. It is common for many generations to live in the same compound, sometimes each in a different house. There are no government social services, and no means-tested pension or other facilities for older adults in general. Nor are there nursing homes of any kind.

The family is entirely responsible for older parents either in health or sickness. Often the first female daughter (locally called Ada), whether married or single, is the principal care provider. The first male child and other children may give some financial or other material support to the Ada but in most cases the mother will move in with the Ada when a chronic disease such as dementia arises. If the Ada is married, her family may have no difficulty accepting her mother (whether the father is alive or not). For fathers who need support, however, it is unusual to move in either with the male children or with the Ada. In such cases, the wife (no matter her age) remains the principal caregiver if a chronic condition should set in. If the wife is dead, the children may as a preference marry the older male to a younger woman or hire a housemaid for him (no matter his age). In general there are more widows than widowers.

Older adults who have no children sometimes have some of their needs met by other extended family members or by some society within the church. The community in general, especially neighbours and religious organizations, are often generous towards older adults and in festival seasons will provide them with valuable gifts.

*Source: Reference 270.*

| 10/66 dementia research group study site | Number | Household living arrangements | | | | Characteristics of the main caregiver | | | |
|---|---|---|---|---|---|---|---|---|---|
| | | Alone (%) | Spouse only (%) | Adult children (%) | One or more children under age 16 (%) | Spouse % | Child or child-in-law (%) | Non-relative (%) | Female caregiver (%) |
| Cuba | 316 | 6.3 | 10.2 | 54.7 | 33.7 | 17.3 | 67.7 | 5.8 | 80.0 |
| Dominican Republic | 235 | 8.5 | 10.2 | 48.5 | 39.9 | 21.4 | 44.6 | 11.6 | 81.3 |
| Venezuela | 140 | 5.7 | 4.9 | 68.1 | 53.8 | 13.7 | 68.4 | 2.8 | 80.7 |
| Peru (urban) | 129 | 1.6 | 9.4 | 54.3 | 27.1 | 13.0 | 41.6 | 30.1 | 83.7 |
| Peru (rural) | 36 | 13.9 | 8.3 | 63.9 | 38.9 | 16.7 | 58.4 | 2.8 | 86.1 |
| Mexico (urban) | 86 | 14.0 | 9.3 | 55.8 | 38.4 | 5.8 | 79.1 | 3.5 | 83.7 |
| Mexico (rural) | 85 | 16.5 | 11.1 | 55.3 | 31.8 | 12.9 | 68.2 | 2.4 | 76.5 |
| China (urban) | 81 | 2.5 | 34.5 | 38.3 | 7.4 | 36.1 | 47.3 | 13.9 | 66.7 |
| China (rural) | 56 | 3.6 | 8.9 | 75.0 | 60.7 | 42.9 | 57.1 | 0 | 35.7 |
| India (urban) | 75 | 4.0 | 13.3 | 72.0 | 49.2 | 26.7 | 40.0 | 0 | 69.3 |
| India (rural) | 10 | 15.1 | 5.7 | 67.0 | 52.8 | 23.3 | 70.0 | 0 | 80.2 |

TABLE 5.1 Household living arrangements and characteristics of the main caregiver for people with dementia at 11 sites in Latin America, China and India. Source: References *3* and *271*.

LMIC country sites one third to two thirds of people with dementia lived in multigenerational households that included children under the age of 16 *(3)* (Table 5.1). Larger households were associated with lesser degrees of caregiver strain *(268)*, probably because care responsibility could be shared and, in principle, the main caregiver could benefit from respite (see the situation in Nigeria in Box 5.1). Demographic, social and economic trends will inevitably impact on the extended family kinship system in LMIC, and the availability and willingness to provide care (see also Chapter 3). Future cohorts of older people may have smaller networks of family caregivers *(269)*.

## WHAT DO FAMILY CAREGIVERS DO?

In the home setting, family caregivers are confronted with multiple tasks that evolve throughout the disease process. Typically, the level of support increases as the disease progresses, starting with support for instrumental activities of daily living (household, financial and social activities) and expanding to include personal care and eventually almost constant supervision. The extent of need and the types of care needed, and their progression over time, depend on many factors such as the clinical profile (types and severity of cognitive impairments and behavioural and psychological symptoms, which may vary by subtype of dementia), the presence of comorbid physical and psychological problems, the custom and habits of the person with dementia, the person's personality and significant relationships. Table 5.2 describes symptoms that commonly affect people with dementia syndrome as the disease progresses from the early stage through to the late stage *(272, 273)*. It shows the probable impact of these impairments on the person with dementia and the changing role of the caregiver. It should be noted that this is a general description of the course of dementia, and that symptomatic features will vary considerably from person to person and within and between the different diseases that result in dementia. The caregiver's role will vary accordingly.

Dementia care is difficult and requires time, energy and, often, physical exertion from the caregiver. As the disease progresses slowly, family members often provide care for many years and are under high levels of stress for long periods of time. The effects of high stress levels are intensified by the chronic fatigue associated with providing long hours of care without periods of relief.

In the late stage, caregivers usually need the assistance of professional care if the person continues living in the community. This is particularly so when caregiving requires significant physical input and when the emotional impact requires respite for caregivers to enable them to continue in their role for as long as possible.

## WHAT ARE THE MOTIVATIONS TO CARE?

Much of the literature on caregiving tends to focus on negative aspects. Strain arises when coping resources are overwhelmed. Therefore, it is important to document that most family and friends involved in providing informal care take pride in their role, and perceive many positives. For some, caring can be rewarding *(274)* and can provide a sense of meaning or self-efficacy *(275)*. In a Canadian study, 80% of a nationally representative sample of caregivers identified positive factors – including companionship (23%), fulfillment (13%), enjoyment (13%), providing quality of life (6%) and meaningfulness (6%) – in association with their role *(3)*.

Affection is a key motivating factor for caregivers of people with dementia *(276)*. In the EUROFAMCARE study, "emotional bonds" (i.e. love and affection) were the principle motivation for providing care, as reported by 57%, followed by a "sense of duty" reported by 15% and a "personal sense of obligation" reported by 13%. Just 3% of caregivers in the study said they "had no other alternative" than to care *(265)*. Another study found that caregiving for a spouse is seen as a natural marital obligation, and that spousal caregivers may report positive feelings toward caregiving *(277)*. In many LMIC, filial obligation or responsibility is reported as being a prime motivator. In such cases the primary caregiver may be designated according to the norms of the particular culture. Reports from Africa suggest that one of the reasons for Africans having many children is that they view children as a form of social security *(278)*. The care provided by the children is sometimes seen not just as a mere duty but as a moral obligation to repay the parents in their old age *(279)*. In a qualitative study carried out in India, seven caregivers felt they were doing their duty by looking after their relative with dementia and six said it was their fate to face such hardships *(280)*.

| Stages of dementia | Common changes experienced by people with dementia | What do caregivers do? |
|---|---|---|
| Early stage | • Become forgetful, especially regarding things that just happened<br>• May have some difficulty with communication, such as difficulty in finding words<br>• Become lost in familiar places<br>• Lose track of the time, including time of day, month, year, season<br>• Have difficulty making decisions and handling personal finances<br>• Have difficulty carrying out complex household tasks<br>• Mood and behaviour:<br>– may become less active and motivated and lose interest in activities and hobbies<br>– may show mood changes, including depression or anxiety<br>– may react unusually angrily or aggressively on occasion. | *Family members become aware of changes and may prompt the person to seek assessment (in pre-diagnostic phase)*<br><br>*Caregivers become aware of their caregiving role (often as a result of diagnosis)*<br><br>• Provide emotional support following diagnosis and when the person is depressed or anxious<br>• Prompt and remind the person about events, tasks and other things to help them maintain involvement and independence<br>• Provide assistance with instrumental activities (e.g. personal finances, shopping). |
| Middle stage | • Become very forgetful, especially of recent events and people's names<br>• Have difficulty comprehending time, date, place and events; may become lost at home as well as in the community<br>• Have increasing difficulty with communication (speech and comprehension)<br>• Need help with personal care (i.e. toileting, washing, dressing)<br>• Unable to successfully prepare food, cook, clean or shop<br>• Unable to live alone safely without considerable support<br>• Behaviour changes may include wandering, repeated questioning, calling out, clinging, disturbed sleeping, hallucinations (seeing or hearing things which are not there)<br>• May display inappropriate behaviour in the home or in the community (e.g. disinhibition, aggression). | *Caregivers become aware of their supervisory role*<br><br>• Use communication strategies to aid understanding<br>• Provide help with carrying out personal care<br>• Provide help with other activities of daily living such as food preparation, dressing appropriately<br>• Respond to and manage behavioural disturbance and inappropriate behaviour. |
| Late stage | • Usually unaware of time and place<br>• Have difficulty understanding what is happening around them<br>• Unable to recognize relatives, friends and familiar objects<br>• Unable to eat without assistance, may have difficulty in swallowing<br>• Increasing need for assisted self-care (bathing and toileting)<br>• May have bladder and bowel incontinence<br>• Change in mobility, may be unable to walk or be confined to a wheelchair or bed<br>• Behaviour changes, may escalate and include aggression towards carer, nonverbal agitation ( kicking, hitting, screaming or moaning)<br>• Unable to find his or her way around in the home. | *Significant demands on caregivers as the care recipient becomes fully dependent and loses the ability to communicate needs and wishes*<br><br>• Provide care, support and supervision around the clock<br>• Provide full assistance with eating and drinking<br>• Provide full physical care (bathing, toileting, dressing, mobilizing)<br>• Manage behavioural problems. |

**TABLE 5.2** Common symptoms experienced by people with dementia syndrome, and activities carried out by caregivers

## WHAT ARE THE CONSEQUENCES OF CAREGIVING?

Those involved in providing services for people with dementia often speak of a second patient in the making (the family caregiver) when a person is diagnosed with dementia *(281)*. This is an important reminder of the need to give equal priority to the needs of the primary caregiver who is a crucial resource in the long-term care arrangements for the person with dementia. Caring for a person with dementia can have a negative effect on the caregiver's psychological *(282, 283)* and physical health *(284)*, life expectancy *(285)*, quality of life and economic security. The disease can have profound and often adverse impacts on family dynamics and role functioning. It is often thought that large intergenerational families in traditional societies cope well with dementia and are relatively immune from caregiver strain. However, the pilot studies of the 10/66 Dementia Research Group in 25 sites in LMIC in Africa, Latin America, China and India revealed levels of caregiver strain as high as those typically seen in European and North American studies *(268)*. The primary stressors identified in western research are sometimes compounded by a profound lack of awareness of the nature of the condition, and stigma and blame consequently attaching to the caregiver. Some of these aspects are illustrated in a narrative from the 10/66 Dementia Research Group pilot study from Anambra, Nigeria, related by a 42-year-old married female caregiver with two children of her own, looking after her mother with dementia *(271)*:

"She always wants to go out of the house. She claims to want to go home. She will pack all her belongings and set for home. At times she searches for her 'babies'. People always gather around when I am dragging her back. I feel very ashamed and people like looking. They think she is mad. My brother hired a housemaid to help me. Because of my mother's stubbornness the maid was beating her a lot. The neighbours reported this so I went and took her to back my house. I don't know what to do. My children are now on holiday, but soon school will start and I am in trouble. I no longer go to market since my mother came to stay with me. At times, I lock her inside the house. I need medicine to cure her. Also other people to help. Still, I feel OK caring for my mother."

## CAREGIVER STRAIN

Caregivers experience multiple demands. The time that they must spend caring, the extent of the need for care, and the variety and intensity of behavioural, cognitive and psychological symptoms that they must address on a daily basis are sometimes referred to as primary stressors *(259)*. Secondary stressors include role strain (e.g. managing the competing demands of child care, work and care for an older relative with dementia) which can lead to suppressed hostility. Family conflict may arise from a lack of shared awareness of the nature of the condition and the extent of the demands placed on the primary caregiver, or from a perception that the caregiving responsibility is not shared, or from disagreements about financial matters relating to care. Caregivers are also at risk of becoming socially isolated because of the demanding nature of their role *(286)*. The stress/health model by Schulz and Martire *(259)* envisages coping resources and external support as modifiers of the effects of primary and secondary stressors on caregiver strain and downstream caregiver morbidity (e.g. adverse psychological and physical health outcomes). When the resources of the caregiver and the wider network are overwhelmed, caregiver strain and morbidity occur.

Previous research has consistently identified caregiver factors, certain clinical features of dementia, and aspects of the premorbid relationship between the caregiver and care recipient as being important determinants of the extent of strain experienced by the caregiver, as highlighted in Table 5.3 *(3)*.

Most of these pathways to caregiver strain and morbidity could be amenable to intervention (Table 5.5), focusing upon education, provision of information, training and psychological and practical support.

Four narratives from caregivers of people with dementia recruited into the 10/66 Dementia Research Group pilot studies from Bangalore, India, illustrate the range of positive and negative caregiver experiences and the role of some of these influences (Box 5.2) *(271)*.

| **The caregiver** | |
|---|---|
| **Caregiver demographic factors** | • Female caregivers<br>• Spousal caregivers, particularly those of younger patients<br>• Caregivers living with the care recipient<br>• Caregivers with low incomes or financial strain |
| **Caregiver personality** | • High level of neuroticism<br>• High expressed emotion |
| **Caregiver perception and experience of caregiving role** | • Low sense of confidence in the role<br>• High "role captivity" (caregivers may feel trapped in the role) |
| **Coping strategies** | • Emotion-based or confrontational coping strategies |
| **The person with dementia** | |
| **Dementia type** | • Frontotemporal dementia |
| **Severity** | • Behavioural and psychological symptoms of dementia (particularly apathy, irritability, anxiety, depression, delusional beliefs)<br>• Cognitive impairment is not usually associated with caregiver strain |
| **Relationship factors** | |
| **Intimacy** | • Poorer relationship quality<br>• Low levels of past and current intimacy |

**TABLE 5.3** Factors related to caregiver strain *(3)*

## PSYCHOLOGICAL IMPACT

Family caregivers of people with dementia are exceptionally prone to affective disorders such as major depression and anxiety disorder *(285, 287)*. A systematic literature search of studies reporting major depressive disorders in caregivers of people with dementia identified 10 studies with a total of 790 caregivers, 176 (22.3%) of whom had a depressive disorder (prevalence range 15–32%) *(287)*. Data on anxiety disorders in dementia caregivers are scarce but suggest that 1 in 3 caregivers suffers from such a disorder *(288)*. Depressive and anxiety symptoms are even more prevalent, affecting between half to three quarters of all caregivers *(287, 289)*. Female caregivers have higher levels of depressive and anxiety symptoms and lower life satisfaction *(290, 291)*. The risk of developing an affective disorder persists over many years of caregiving and even after caregiving ends with the death of a care recipient *(285, 292)*.

Pilot studies in 24 of the 10/66 Dementia Research Group study centres in Africa, Latin America, and South and South-East Asia revealed that the levels of psychological morbidity among 706 caregivers of people with dementia were at least as high as those seen in high-income countries *(268)*. In the same study, the presence of behavioural and psychological symptoms of dementia in the care recipient was strongly associated with caregiver strain *(271)*. The caregivers reported strain associated with managing behavioural and psychological symptoms of dementia from a variety of sources, the physical and emotional strain of providing care with inadequate support from other family members, and the financial strain consequent on having to cut back on work in order to care.

BOX 5.2

## VOICES OF CAREGIVERS FROM INDIA

**Caregiver 1**
**(a 28-year-old married man, looking after his father)**
Sometimes he forgets our names; that is what is difficult. Otherwise there is no problem in looking after him. That at such an age he should have this problem is painful for us. Everybody understands his problem. Family and friends are very helpful. They come over frequently and give us advice as to what we should do. Right now there isn't much work for us. My wife and I manage to look after him. He has looked after us, his children, so well for all these years. It gives me pleasure to look after him. God has given me an opportunity to serve him.

**Caregiver 2**
**(a 23-year-old married woman, with two children, caring for a distant relative)**
Her wandering behaviour, picking up objects from the road, and her urine incontinence. It is difficult to take care of her because of these things. Somebody has to be with her all the time. People are very supportive. We can visit anyone's house with her and people also come and visit us. If she wanders away somewhere there are enough people to bring her back. Neighbours, other family members, everybody is supportive of us. No help is needed. We are her children. What else can we do but look after her?

**Caregiver 3**
**(48-year-old unmarried woman, caring for her father)**
We find it difficult to socialize. Calling people home is difficult. He doesn't sleep throughout the night. He is incontinent; mother has to look after him. He often slips away. Family members think we are the cause of his illness; they think we deserve all that is happening to us. Other than our family, we don't really know or care how others feel about him. We can look after him for now. My mother is not very comfortable (asking for help) as people will blame her for my father's problems. It is better not to ask anybody. Obviously we would like it if there was paid help but right now it isn't an option, mainly because my mother refuses to let anyone else help him. We feel it's a burden. As a father or a husband we haven't got anything from him all these years and now we have to look after him.

**Caregiver 4**
**(55-year-old married woman, caring for her father)**
He quarrels with me, uses bad language, beats me, runs away from home and I have to catch him. He behaves like a mad person. People say to me that he is mad, and tell me to take him to the hospital. The children don't understand about his problems. No one is there to help me. My children help me a little. If someone could help us with money, that would be nice. There is no one else to look after him. I only have to do it. No one else can help. I don't feel angry, there's no point. I have to do it.

*Source: Reference 271.*

## IMPACT ON PHYSICAL HEALTH

Caregivers of people with dementia self-report poorer health outcomes, lower subjective well-being scores, and poorer quality of life than non-caregivers. They also experience worse health outcomes, including obesity, higher metabolic risk *(293)*, higher levels of stress hormones, compromised immune response, antibodies, greater medication use and greater cognitive decline *(293, 294)*.

Schulz and Martire *(259)* conducted a review of the health effects of being a caregiver for a person with dementia. They found research showing reduced engagement in preventive health behaviours *(295)*, decreased immunity *(296–298)*, greater cardiovascular reactivity *(299)*, and slower wound healing *(300)*. Evidence also suggests that caregivers may be at increased risk for serious illness *(297, 301)* and mortality *(285)*.

## ECONOMIC IMPACT

Providing dementia care can become a full-time job without adequate support. Caregivers may be forced to quit work, cut back on work, or take a less demanding job in order to provide care.

In USA in 2010, nearly 15 million family and other unpaid caregivers provided an estimated 17 billion hours of care to people with dementia, a contribution valued at more than US$ 202 billion *(302)*. The global economic impact of caregiving for dementia has been estimated in detail, based on a systematic review of the world literature, for the *World Alzheimer Report 2010 (7)*. A summary table on informal care inputs (hours per day) is presented in Table 5.4. Where estimates were not available for a particular world region they were imputed from findings from a neighbouring region with similar characteristics. The caregiver time was quantified as:

| GBD region (green = imputed) | Basic ADL | Combined ADL | Supervision |
|---|---|---|---|
| Australasia | 2.0 | 3.3 | 2.6 |
| Asia Pacific, High Income | 2.0 | 3.6 | 2.6 |
| Oceania | 3.6 | 4.6 | 1.2 |
| Asia, Central | 1.2 | 2.7 | 3.3 |
| Asia, East | 3.6 | 4.7 | 1.2 |
| Asia, South | 1.3 | 2.7 | 2.6 |
| Asia, South-East | 1.3 | 2.7 | 2.6 |
| Europe, Western | 1.1 | 3.5 | 3.3 |
| Europe, Central | 2.1 | 4.4 | 3.4 |
| Europe, Eastern | 2.1 | 4.4 | 3.4 |
| North America, High Income | 2.1 | 4.0 | 2.8 |
| Caribbean | 3.0 | 3.0 | 2.1 |
| Latin America, Andean | 2.9 | 2.9 | 2.6 |
| Latin America, Central | 1.9 | 1.9 | 3.1 |
| Latin America, Southern | 2.9 | 4.4 | 2.6 |
| Latin America, Tropical | 2.9 | 2.9 | 2.6 |
| North Africa/Middle East | 1.0 | 1.4 | 2.8 |
| Sub-Saharan Africa, Central | 2.0 | 3.6 | 2.6 |
| Sub-Saharan Africa, East | 2.0 | 3.6 | 2.6 |
| Sub-Saharan Africa, Southern | 2.0 | 3.6 | 2.6 |
| Sub-Saharan Africa, West | 2.0 | 3.6 | 2.6 |
| **All** | **2.0** | **3.6** | **2.6** |

TABLE 5.4 Global Burden of Disease region-specific figures of informal care inputs (hours per day) *(7)*

- assistance with basic ADL, such as eating, dressing, bathing, toileting, grooming, and getting around (sometimes referred to as personal care);
- assistance with combined ADL, including also IADL, such as shopping, preparing food, using transport, and managing personal finances;
- supervision to manage behavioural symptoms or to prevent dangerous events.

Table 5.4 shows that caregivers spend 3.6 hours per day on average assisting with activities of daily living (basic ADL + IADL care inputs).

## INTERVENTIONS FOR CAREGIVERS

The accumulating evidence on the personal, social and health impacts of caregiving has generated intervention studies aimed at decreasing the stress of caregiving.

The dominant theoretical model guiding the design of caregiver interventions is the stress/health model *(259)*. According to the model, primary stressors on the caregiver depend on the degree of cognitive impairment of the person with dementia, the frequency of problem behaviours by the care recipient, the number of hours per week required to provide physical assistance, and the need to navigate the health care system. Secondary stressors on the caregiver, which may be less obvious to care providers, include missed work opportunities and family conflict. Both primary and secondary stressors may lead to perceived stress and ultimately morbidity or mortality. The model thus recommends a multi-faceted intervention scheme for caregivers. This includes a focus on the person with dementia so primary stressors can be reduced (e.g. reduction of disruptive behaviours), caregiver knowledge regarding social support and resource availability so adaptive capacities can be bolstered, and approaches to caregiver behaviour so behavioural responses to stressors can be improved.

Many studies, mainly conducted in high-income countries, attest to the wide-ranging benefits of caregiver interventions. There are several systematic reviews and meta-analyses *(283, 303–307)*. A recent review evaluated the evidence on the efficacy and effectiveness of psychological and psychosocial interventions *(307)*. These studies cover a wide range of intervention programmes such as caregiver information and education, psycho-educational training (e.g. for self-management of moods), training in coping skills (e.g. implementing assistive technologies), support groups, counselling for primary caregivers and family (face-to-face, telephone or videolink), psychotherapy (e.g. cognitive behaviour therapy), respite and multi-component studies. The review concluded that non-pharmacological treatments "emerge as a useful, versatile, and potentially cost-effective approach to improve outcomes and quality of life for both the person with dementia and caregiver". Table 5.5 lists brief descriptions of the types of intervention considered.

Although the effects are generally moderate and variable, several studies have shown that interventions can have a positive effect on caregiver strain, depression and subjective well-being *(283, 304, 329, 330)*, with psychoeducational interventions having the greatest effect on reducing depression in one review *(283)*. Interventions may play an important and helpful part in mitigating distress in some caregivers. They are likely to be most effective when they are initiated after careful evaluation of the caregivers' needs, resources and ability to access existing services *(331)*, and with careful attention to how service needs vary across the continuum of dementia decline.

| Interventions | Brief description | Key citations |
|---|---|---|
| Individual and family counselling | Individual and family counselling provided by trained providers for treatment of caregiver depression and managing stress. Ad hoc telephone access also available. | References 308–312 |
| Psychoeducational programmes [1], e.g.:<br>• Coping with Caregiving<br>• Savvy Caregiving | Caregivers are taught a set of behavioural and cognitive skills for coping with caregiving demands and stress, using a structural format. | References 307, 314–317 |
| Specialized skill trainings, e.g.:<br>• Behaviour Management<br>• STAR-C (Staff Training in Assisted-living Residences-Caregivers)<br>• In-Home Modifications | Training focuses on a specific issue related to caregiving, such as home modifications, managing difficult behaviours and dealing with the frustrations of the person with dementia, managing sleep disruption, and promotion of exercises to alleviate stress. | References 318–324 |
| Multicomponent programmes (i.e. REACH II (Resources for Enhancing Alzheimer's Caregiver Health II)) [2] | A multicomponent programme that consists of home visits to create individualized plans for caregivers to manage their stress, behavioural interventions, telephone support group calls, and access to various local resources. | References 325, 326 |
| Psychotherapy/cognitive behavioural therapy | Use of cognitive behavioural therapy to treat caregivers who are clinically depressed or who have other significant mental health problems. | References 327, 328 |

[1] Psychoeducational and/or behaviour management training programmes have been used in the Australia, India, Spain, United Kingdom and some other parts of Europe. Work is ongoing in other regions of the world (e.g. China, Hong Kong Special Administrative Region).

[2] Adaptations of REACH II are currently in dissemination trials in many parts of the USA.

**TABLE 5.5** Examples of effective interventions for family caregivers

The beneficial effects of caregiver interventions on institutionalization of the care recipient have been clearly and directly demonstrated. In their meta-analysis, Brodaty et al *(304)* concluded that caregiver interventions could delay nursing home admission. Interventions which involved the person with dementia and those which were multicomponent were more likely to be successful. A systematic review of 10 randomized controlled trials has indicated a 40% reduction in the pooled odds of institutionalization *(306)*. The effective interventions were structured, intensive and multicomponent, offering a choice of services and supports to caregivers *(283, 306)*. The Mittelman trial observed a greater benefit as regards institutionalization when the interventions were started earlier in the disease course *(310)*. Interventions that help reduce nursing home utilization without increasing caregiver strain are important for achieving the move towards quality community focused care in high-income countries.

Financial benefit from interventions that delay institutionalization have also been measured. A USA-based cost-benefit analysis of earlier diagnosis of Alzheimer's Disease, treatment with acetylcholinestrase inhibitors and provision of caregiver interventions showed that early intervention can delay institutionalization and potentially reduce health care costs. The net benefits were highest in cases that were identified in the earlier stage of dementia and where caregiver intervention programmes were implemented.

An important issue is the effectiveness of interventions in caregivers from diverse ethnic, racial, cultural and linguistic backgrounds. Most of the above programmes have been used only in high-income countries, and some have not been used outside the USA, although a culturally-tailored version of the REACH programme has been conducted in a controlled study in China, Hong Kong Special Administrative Region (Hong Kong SAR) *(332)*. Another study suggests that psychosocial intervention of demonstrated effectiveness might be made available cheaply in LMIC since they are typically of low cost (the cost being chiefly related to the human effort involved) *(307)*.

Some literature is available from LMIC on caregiver interventions. Dias et al. *(235)* reported on the effectiveness of the *Helping Carers to Care* home care programme for dementia caregivers in Goa, India (Box 4.9). In this study, the community-based intervention was provided by a team consisting of home care advisers who were supervised by a counsellor and a psychiatrist. The intervention focused on supporting the caregiver by providing information on dementia, guidance on behaviour management, a single psychiatric assessment and psychotropic medication if needed. The strain on caregivers was much reduced and the mental health of the caregivers improved. The study concluded that home-based support for caregivers of persons with dementia, which emphasizes the use of locally available, low-cost human resources, is feasible, acceptable and leads to significant improvements in caregiver mental health and burden of caring. Researchers from the 10/66 Dementia Research Group have since tested the effectiveness of this intervention in randomized controlled trials in Peru and Russia *(201, 236, 238)*. The results again indicated much larger treatment effects on caregiver psychological morbidity and strain than are typically seen in trials of such interventions in high-income countries.

There are also forthcoming examples of services and infrastructure that are planned to support patients with dementia and their family caregivers in China, including the Hong Kong SAR and the Province of Taiwan *(333)*. In these Chinese societies, although children and family are still thought to be the most reliable sources of caregiving for a family member with dementia, the need for more public resources is acknowledged as the traditional belief in filial piety is increasingly eroded. Thompson et al. recommends that policy-makers and service planners require more data that address questions such as: "How is this service likely to be most beneficial?" and "At what stage in the caregiving process should this service be introduced for maximum effectiveness?" *(334)*. It is important that interventions take place along the continuum of care from initial diagnosis through to end-of-life care. A key issue is that, despite quite convincing evidence of effectiveness, there have been no successful examples of scale-up in any of the health systems in which the evaluative research has been conducted. Further research should focus on implementation in order to inform the process of scale-up, identifying and addressing barriers and providing further evidence of cost-effectiveness.

**BOX 5.3**

## CARER'S STRATEGY FOR MAURITIUS

The Republic of Mauritius launched a *Carer's Strategy* and Action Plan (CSAP) in January 2010.

Mauritius has 156 700 elderly people in a population of 1.3 million (i.e. 12.7% of the total population). It is estimated that the percentage will increase to 20% by the year 2040. Life expectancy is currently 70 years for males and 78 years for females. With the phenomenon of ageing and the advent of the industrial economy, the number of people requiring care for disability is increasing.

The CSAP aims to create a pool of some 1 000 formal caregivers over a period of five years and to provide the necessary training to some 25 000 informal caregivers who are presently beneficiaries of the carer's allowance from the Ministry of Social Security, National Solidarity and Reform Institutions.

The specific objectives of the *Carer's Strategy* are:

1. To create a pool of formally trained caregivers, to respond to the demand for paid carers by families who are providing care to loved ones;
2. To provide basic training to informal caregivers to enable them to provide better quality care to members of their families;
3. To provide respite care services to informal caregivers to enable them to participate in educational, social and community programmes;
4. To enable informal caregivers to balance employment needs with their care role in the family;
5. To provide a platform for caregivers to express their views in decision-making.

The strategy is accompanied by a five-year action plan.

The ministry and the Mauritius Institute of Health have started the training of formal caregivers with a nine-month training programme comprising both theory and practice. Work-based placements are undertaken at a specialized centre for older people with severe disabilities.

The Ministry's Medical Unit is organizing around 10 training courses annually for informal caregivers. Each of the three-day courses is attended by some 50 participants.

A monitoring mechanism has been set up by the various stakeholders (ministries, employers association, NGOs and others) to monitor progress made and to ensure that the CSAP is being implemented.

It appears that there is increasing professionalization of formal caregivers. This could be an important source of employment for persons who are appropriately motivated and compassionate.

*Source: Reference 349.*

## ADVANCES IN COMMUNICATIONS AND ASSISTIVE TECHNOLOGIES

A range of intervention approaches using communication technology has been empirically studied and found to be helpful to improve the quality of life of family caregivers of people with dementia. The most frequently used and studied are telephones and videophones used by professional practitioners for counselling and support services (335). Video-based psychoeducation intervention has also demonstrated improvements in the mental health of caregivers, including lower levels of stress *(336)*.

The rapidly increasing availability of the internet also offers a potential avenue for support. It may be an appropriate technology for accessing evidence-based treatment programmes such as cognitive behaviour therapy. Another potential source from the internet is in social media networks which can enable networking between caregivers and increased access to information from a variety of sources, although reliability could be an issue. Recently established virtual communities such as PatientsLikeMe, QuitNet and CureTogether are also fertile ground for family caregivers who are motivated to seek their own sources of information.

Assistive technologies are tools that can be used to maintain independent living, improve the safety and autonomy of people with dementia, and support their quality of life by enhancing their peace of mind and that of their family caregivers *(335, 337, 338)*. Examples include alarm sensors to prevent individuals from wandering away, sensors to turn off gas or stove, and pill dispensers that tweet, text or e-mail caregivers if pills are not taken at the appropriate time. The list will become longer as technologies advance.

Innovative technology such as internet can make evidence-based interventions and other programmes and services more readily available and accessible to benefit caregivers wherever they may live. Disparities exist in terms of access and distribution of such programmes, however, especially for caregivers in rural and remote areas, in LMIC, and from ethnic minority populations *(339)*. While technology may help to meet needs and provide essential information *(337, 339, 340)*, the need for skilled assistance in supporting caregivers should not be ignored.

In their systematic review of technologies supporting family caregivers, Powell and colleagues concluded that, although there are many positive findings, on balance this literature should be interpreted cautiously *(341)*. Effects were found to vary considerably among caregivers with different characteristics (e.g. initial level of burden). More research and evaluation in programme settings needs to be done to assess the benefit and cost-effectiveness of the use of technology *(338)*.

## UTILIZATION OF CAREGIVER INTERVENTIONS: KEY ISSUES

In high-income countries and in regions within countries that are more affluent, programmes involving highly skilled professional staff may be feasible and scalable. In contrast, in many areas of LMIC, programmes like the 10/66 programme described above which use non-specialized health and social care professionals who have been given specialized skill training, may be more practical and therefore more likely to be used.

Generally, researchers and service providers agree on several key elements associated with the utilization of caregiver interventions.

- In order to evaluate clearly the needs, strengths, weaknesses and available resources, it is highly recommended that a comprehensive assessment should be done before any services are recommended, and the results of the assessment should be used to guide the selection of intervention.

- The programme staff/assessor must be familiar with the services and resources available in the particular area, with the eligibility criteria for caregivers, and with the cost (if any) so that appropriate referrals can be made.

- If the programme is comprehensive and offers a wide range of services, then trained staff must be present to deliver the interventions.

- The outcomes of the intervention should be measured, and preferably at frequent intervals, so that adjustments can be made if no progress is seen.

- Interventions should allow for flexibility in how they are implemented so that they can be tailored to the specific needs of each caregiver, which may be quite distinct.

Despite evidence of the efficacy of caregiver interventions, funding for research to scale up these approaches is limited. Although finding more effective treatments for dementia is essential for future disease control, providing support for those currently living with the disease and their families is also vital.

## BARRIERS TO ACCESSING CAREGIVER SERVICES

The barriers to accessing caregiver support services are the same as those identified for accessing dementia-appropriate health and social services in general. These barriers include negative attitudes to diagnosis and treatment, lack of appropriately trained health workforce and of the infrastructure to scale up services, low help-seeking because dementia is considered part of normal ageing or because of stigma, lack of public policy initiatives, and lack of funds for dementia services, research, and training.

Caregivers also face additional barriers when seeking services for themselves. In many LMIC, no support services are routinely available for family caregivers. Even in high-income countries there are barriers to access and uptake, including lack of recognition of the caregiving role, poor understanding of dementia and cultural influences on caregiving.

### ROLE RECOGNITION

Family members often do not consider themselves caregivers, so they do not look for services that can support them in that role. Those who seek such services often find them to be scattered, uncoordinated and not appropriate to their needs *(342)*. Health insurance policies often do not provide coverage for caregiver support services. Along with fragmented care systems, lack of knowledge about resources, and the emotional burdens of care provision, caregivers for people with dementia encounter the stigmatization of the disease. Caregivers and policy-makers alike need to recognize the importance and dignity of the caregiver role.

### LACK OF KNOWLEDGE

Poor literacy, including dementia literacy, also contributes to lack of access to services *(343–346)*. The range of skills required for adequate health literacy (e.g. understanding medical terminology and information clearly enough to be able to follow directions, recognize and respond appropriately to symptoms) are developed over a lifetime. When caregivers' health literacy is low, their attitudes and behaviour are affected.

### CULTURAL APPROACHES TO CAREGIVING

In most Asian cultures that have been studied (such as Chinese, Korean and Malaysian), it is common for families to take full responsibility for older adults with dementia. This may be coupled with a reluctancy to discuss dementia and related caregiving issues with people outside the immediate family due to fears of "losing face". This often results in refusal of outside help even when it is likely to be much needed *(345–347)*. This approach to coping results in less social and emotional support for caregivers. It part of a vicious circle whereby being unable to acknowledge the disease for what it is leads to an inability to access services.

## STRENGTHENING CAREGIVING

Given the important role of caregivers, both in maintaining the quality of life of the care recipient and in providing the most cost-effective model of long-term care, appropriate and accessible support structures are vital.

A three-fold approach to strengthen caregiving includes:

- **Information, resources and training:** Information needs include understanding the characteristics and course of the disease and what resources are available to families, along with training in how to care for people with the disease and how to prevent and deal with behavioural symptoms.

- **Support and respite:** There are a number of strategies for supporting caregivers, including counselling and long-term support, dyadic interventions, caregiver retreats, respite care (described in chapter 4), and family meetings that include the person with dementia. It is urgent to implement strategies that are successful and replicable, focusing on both best practices and promising ones.

- **Financial support:** Caregivers need financial assistance in order to do their jobs well and to sustain them for the long term. A few models are in place worldwide such as the long-term care insurance in Japan (Box 3.6). In addition to caregiver benefits, disability benefits for the person with dementia and social pensions also have a part to play, as described in chapter 3.

None of the steps, however, is simple. Cultural factors, linguistic issues and health literacy concerns must be considered when educating family and friends about dementia and care options. These issues are more commonly found in LMIC, although ethnic and racial minorities in high-income countries face similar challenges *(348)*.

The predicted future shortage of human resource capacity must also be addressed, alongside an expansion of services that are known to be effective and culturally appropriate and that are likely to be accessed. Given the insufficient number of specialists in LMIC, dementia care will require the engagement of community health workers, primary care doctors and nurses and family caregivers all working as a team. This will necessitate a pathway to care and support that improves access and communication and that is flexible and adaptable to the changing needs of people with dementia and their caregivers *(158)*. The Republic of Mauritius, as one example, has recently launched a caregiver's strategy to support both formal and informal caregivers (Box 5.3).

## SUMMARY POINTS

- Most care for people with dementia is provided by informal, unpaid caregivers who include spouses, adult children, daughters- and sons-in-law and friends. Women are far more likely to be the caregivers in all countries. However, changing population demographics may reduce the availability of informal caregivers.

- The provision of care to a person with dementia can result in significant strain for those who provide most of that care. The stressors include physical, emotional and economic pressures. Support is needed to enable informal caregivers to continue in their role for as long as possible. Support includes information to aid understanding, skills to assist in caring, respite to enable engagement in other activities, and financial support.

- A range of programmes and services have been developed in high-income countries to assist family caregivers and to reduce strain. However, research on their effectiveness in different social, cultural and geographical contexts is limited. There is an urgent need to develop and implement an array of low-cost or no-cost government-supported services within an accessible infrastructure, so that even those with significant barriers to accessing services will be able to do so if motivated.

- Information and education campaigns for the public – including people with dementia, their caregivers and families – aimed at raising awareness, improving understanding and decreasing stigmatizing attitudes should help overcome barriers to accessing and using services.

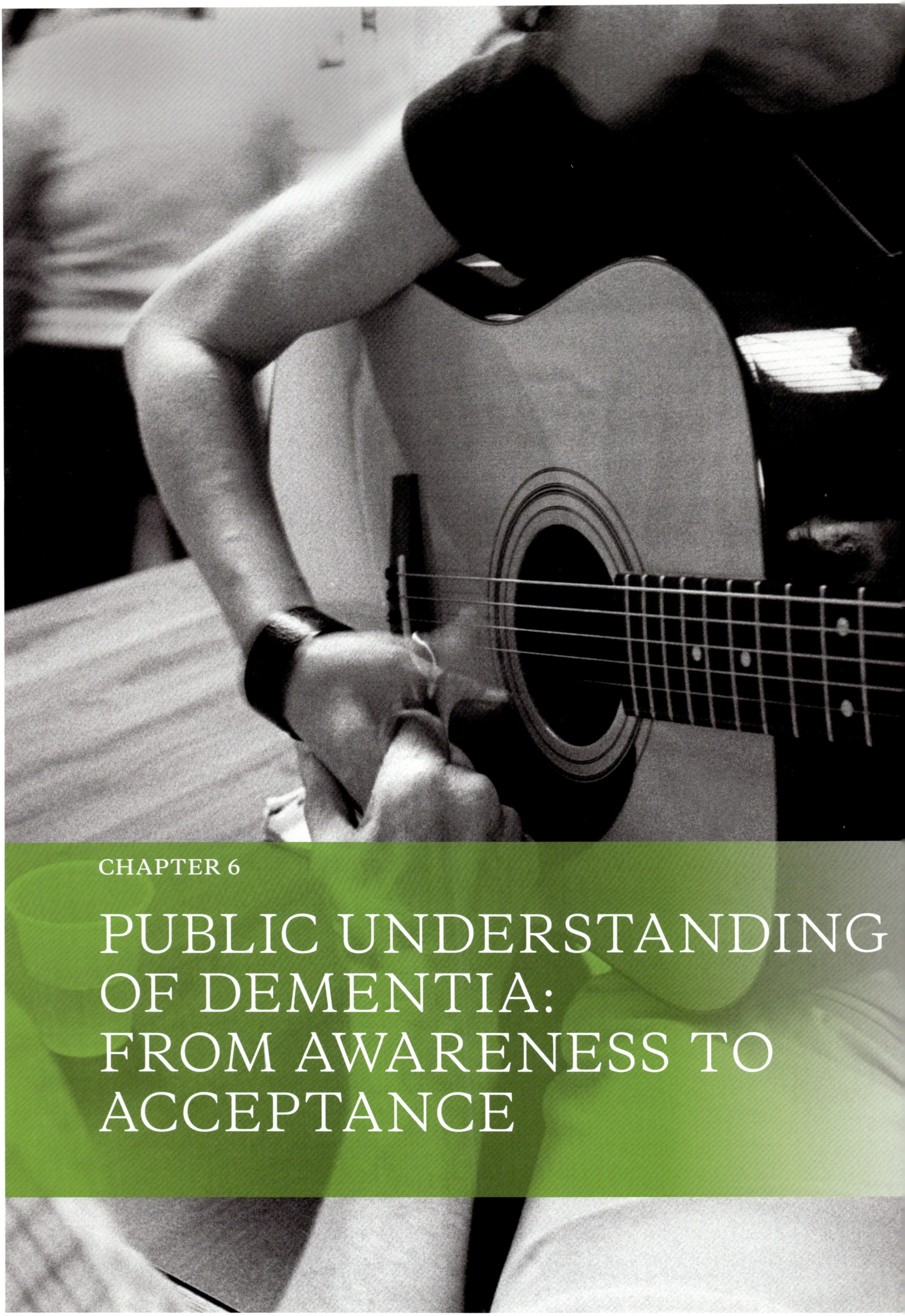

CHAPTER 6

# PUBLIC UNDERSTANDING OF DEMENTIA: FROM AWARENESS TO ACCEPTANCE

Many people know someone affected by dementia. However, despite rising awareness of dementia, understanding of the syndrome is low *(350)*. Dementia is often considered to be a natural part of ageing. Sometimes the symptoms are misunderstood as being caused by evil spirits.

The lack of understanding contributes to fears about developing dementia and fosters stigmatizing practices such as avoidance or discrimination. For those who have dementia and for their caregivers and families, the stigma contributes to social isolation and to delays in seeking a diagnosis and help.

This chapter examines awareness, knowledge and attitudes to dementia within society. It is imperative that public awareness and understanding is enhanced in order to reduce the stigma associated with dementia and to enable people with dementia and their caregivers to access support at the appropriate time. Processes for supporting a move towards acceptance of dementia are outlined and illustrated with examples of public and political campaigns to support a societal shift towards acceptance and inclusion of dementia and the people who are affected by it.

## AWARENESS AND UNDERSTANDING OF DEMENTIA

Several themes emerge from the literature relating to the lack of awareness and understanding of dementia among the public *(351)*. First, it is often understood to be a normal part of ageing rather than a disease process.

Second, people do not know about or recognize the symptoms of dementia. For example, 81% of respondents of the "Facing Dementia Survey" conducted in Europe believed that most people do not know the difference between the early stages of Alzheimer's disease and behaviour associated with normal ageing *(352)*.

Finally, there is a lack of understanding of the associated risk factors. As vascular risk factors (including hypertension and high cholesterol) are also likely to be risk factors for dementia, an understanding of this link can encourage lifestyle modifications.

A number of statements on awareness and understanding of dementia in their country were put to the WHO dementia survey respondents. There was a marked difference in responses between high-income and LMIC. There is a greater likelihood that dementia will be understood as "being due to irreversible and progressive diseases of the brain" in high-income countries, while "no or limited awareness of the syndrome" is more likely in LMIC (Table 6.1). Two respondents also indicated a difference in understanding between city-dwellers and people living in rural and remote areas.

| In your opinion, how do people in general perceive or understand dementia in the country? | High-income countries N=8 | LMIC N=22 |
|---|---|---|
| There is no or limited awareness of the syndrome of dementia or the diseases associated with dementia | 3 (37.5%) | 19 (86.3%) |
| Symptoms of dementia are perceived as a normal part of ageing | 6 (75.0%) | 19 (86.3%) |
| Symptoms of dementia are perceived as a sign on mental illness | 5 (62.5%) | 18 (81.8%) |
| The causes of symptoms of dementia are perceived as being metaphysical (e.g.linked to supernatural or spiritual beliefs) | 0 (0.0%) | 7 (31.8%) |
| There is an understanding of dementia being due to irreversible and progressive diseases of the brain | 7 (87.5%) | 12 (54.5%) |

**TABLE 6.1** WHO dementia survey: Country responses to questions on perception and understanding of dementia

## THE IMPACT OF STIGMA

Low levels of understanding about dementia contribute to a number of misperceptions about the disease and result in a perpetuation of stigma which is, sadly, prevalent in most countries. Misperception occurs on a number of levels: the broader community, people with dementia and their families, and those who provide health and social services to them.

### PUBLIC PERCEPTIONS OF DEMENTIA

Lack of understanding of the nature of the condition in the general public contributes to a fear of developing dementia.

In the *Value of Knowing* study *(353)* conducted by Harvard School of Public Health and Alzheimer Europe in five countries (France, Germany, Poland, Spain and USA) 70% of respondents knew or had known someone with Alzheimer's disease and 30% reported they had a family member with dementia.

Despite this exposure, findings indicate that dementia is the biggest health fear after cancer in four of the five countries *(354)*. Similarly, the IMPACT (Important Perspectives on Alzheimer's Care and Treatment) study found that Alzheimer's disease was ranked second out of 10 diseases that people would be most fearful of developing in the future *(355)*.

Results from the IMPACT study indicated that participants were "somewhat concerned" (40.8% of 1 000) or "very concerned" (31.8% of 1 000) about losing contact with family and friends. This fear is reinforced by the negative or derogatory language that may be used to describe people with dementia. In Japan, where the word for dementia has a negative association, the government officially changed the word for the condition (Box 6.1).

Participants in the WHO dementia survey were asked about stigma. Twenty-five of the 30 country respondents indicated that stigma associated with dementia negatively affects people with dementia and family caregivers. Ten respondents explained that people with dementia were isolated or hidden because of shame or because of the potential for behavioural or psychological symptoms to be seen by others.

Socioeconomic and cultural variables contribute to shaping knowledge and beliefs about dementia *(357, 358)*. In LMIC, poor recognition and lack of public awareness cause significant problems *(359)*. Cultural factors such as belief systems influence understanding of and attitudes to dementia. In Togo, for example, symptoms of dementia may be understood as resulting from witchcraft (Box 6.2).

### PERCEPTIONS HELD BY PEOPLE WITH DEMENTIA AND THEIR CAREGIVERS

People with dementia report that they find it difficult to talk about the disease because they fear the consequences which could include loss of friendships *(361)*. A belief that nothing can be done leads to feelings of hopelessness which can affect people's well-being *(362)*.

Stigma and discrimination extend to family caregivers *(363, 364)*. For example, the symptoms experienced by people with dementia, which may include poor self-care or incontinence, are often regarded by others as evidence of neglect *(365)*. Furthermore, to the extent that individuals attempt to avoid social interactions with people with dementia, family caregivers may be inadvertently excluded as well.

**BOX 6.1**

### 10 YEAR NATIONWIDE PROGRAMME IN JAPAN

The word for dementia in Japanese "Chihō" has a negative association. "Chi" means foolishness, and "hō" means dumb or disoriented. It contributes to stigma and fails to show dignity and respect for people with dementia. Therefore, at the end of 2004, the Japanese government changed the word for dementia from "Chihō" to "Ninchishō", which means "disease of cognition". The government has changed all administrative terms to the new word, and the media and academic groups have also accepted the new term.

At the same time, the government launched a 10-year nationwide campaign to raise public awareness and understanding of dementia.

At the heart of the campaign is the "Nationwide caravan to train one million 'Ninchishō (Dementia) Supporters'". In this campaign, specialized seminars for the general public are held all around the country. With greater understanding of the disease and its impact, attendees are expected to become Ninchishō Supporters and advocates for people living with dementia.

By March 2011, over 2.4 million people in Japan had attended the seminars and had become Ninchishō Supporters. They include young people, police officers and people from all backgrounds. After seven years, the new term "Ninchishō" is used widely in Japan and people understand the disease better, resulting in less stigma.

*Source: Reference 356.*

**BOX 6.2**

### TOGO: STIGMA AND MISUNDERSTANDING AROUND DEMENTIA

Dementia is a public health and human rights concern in Togo because of the stigma and misunderstanding which negatively affect people with dementia.

The symptoms of dementia are sometimes understood to be metaphysical. In many Togolese communities a person with dementia who become disorientated is considered to be a witch and is mistreated, hit, or even burned. People with dementia may be sent to convents or to prayer centres to be exorcized.

Until recently, the Togolese health policies were directed primarily to maternal and child health and infectious diseases. There was no official dementia policy. However, today there is growing awareness among public health professionals of the issues relating to dementia in Togo. With impetus from the global action on noncommunicable diseases, mental health, including dementia, is being taken into account in the development of the first NCD policy and strategic plan (2012–2015) of Togo.

*Source: Reference 360.*

### ATTITUDES OF SERVICE PROVIDERS

A few studies have reported that people with dementia have found some general practitioners unhelpful or dismissive about dementia and their symptoms *(366)*. An unhelpful attitude from a service provider, clearly contributes to negative perceptions held by persons living with dementia.

Stigma and misunderstanding can have a devastating impact on all stages of a person's journey through dementia, thus demonstrating the need for urgent action to reduce stigma and to raise the level of understanding across all sectors of society.

## AWARENESS-RAISING CAMPAIGNS

For awareness-raising to be effective, the issues to be addressed must be clearly identified. For example, in the United Kingdom an extensive review of qualitative and quantitative surveys has identified several themes *(351)*. These are:

- raising public awareness and understanding of dementia;
- reducing the stigma of dementia and challenging discriminatory behaviour;
- recognizing the early signs of dementia to aid early diagnosis;
- living well with dementia;
- the importance of a healthy lifestyle and reducing risk.

Similar themes also emerged from the WHO survey. Examples of campaigns and other means of raising awareness according to the five identified themes are described below.

### THEME 1: RAISING PUBLIC AWARENESS AND UNDERSTANDING OF DEMENTIA

At the heart of awareness-raising and information is the message that dementia is a disease causing disability and not an inevitable consequence of ageing. Awareness-raising and understanding are important for countering the fatalism and stigma that is often associated with dementia. They may also contribute to the capacity of family caregivers to cope better with looking after relatives with dementia.

There are many examples of campaigns from around the world that aim to raise awareness and understanding of the condition. The 10-year nationwide campaign undertaken in Japan to raise public awareness and understanding is one such example. It is a large-scale campaign initiated by the government and targeting people from all walks of life, including children (Box 6.1).

Civil society has a major role to play in awareness-raising campaigns. These campaigns often involve celebrities and, more recently, people with dementia and their caregivers who provide a positive image of living with dementia. A global focus for awareness-raising is World Alzheimer Day (21 September) and World Alzheimer's Month (September), which was started by ADI in 1994 and has become an annual day in many countries of the world. A number of examples of activities are provided on the ADI web site *(367)*.

There are few examples of campaigns in LMIC, and still fewer of their effectiveness. One example is the evaluation of responses to the use of a well-known celebrity for a television campaign by the Brazilian Alzheimer Association. The association secured television time and involved a famous actress. The purpose of the campaign was to increase general awareness and, as a result, the number of calls to the helpline rose from 1 000 to 2 400 per month *(368)*.

## THEME 2: REDUCING THE STIGMA OF DEMENTIA

The United Kingdom campaign "I have dementia, I also have a life" demonstrates a targeted approach to dispelling fears in one specific group within society. Targeting a 40–60-year-old predominantly female audience, the campaign – which used television, radio, the press and internet – featured people with dementia. The advertising, which aimed to raise levels of understanding, was developed as a result of qualitative research. Although in previous research people with dementia and their families said they felt stigmatized, the results of the qualitative research, which was conducted with people who had little or no experience of dementia, showed that what was being perceived as stigma was something very different. It showed great fear of dementia, fear of getting the condition and fear of engaging with people with dementia. The advertising campaign therefore sought to "normalize" dementia rather than to "medicalize" it since the latter could lead to increased fear *(369)* (Box 6.3).

## THEME 3: RECOGNIZING THE EARLY SYMPTOMS TO AID IN TIMELY DIAGNOSIS AND INITIATION OF TREATMENT

Many people are not aware of the range of symptoms associated with dementia. They are most likely to view memory loss as a symptom of dementia, rather than other symptoms such as loss of interest or behavioural changes. When people with symptoms, or their families, believe that memory loss is a natural part of ageing they fail to seek medical advice. The health profession has a role to play in this area by actively assessing for symptoms in ageing patients and by providing information to at-risk patients. This is important for raising the awareness of both the general public and the health professionals. The Alzheimer's Association in the USA carried out the "Know the 10 Signs" campaign to raise awareness about the early diagnosis of dementia *(370)*.

## THEME 4: PROMOTING QUALITY OF LIFE

Different media channels such as film, television, internet and social media provide opportunities for disseminating positive images and messages about dementia. The documentary film *I remember better when I paint,* for example, sends a powerful message about the abilities that can remain despite the diagnosis *(371)*.

It also demonstrates the value of activities that provide outlets for expression for people with dementia *(372)*. Although the empirical evidence is not strong *(307)*, some research evidence suggests that engagement in creative arts can provide meaningful stimulation, improve social interaction and improve levels of self-esteem *(373)*.

**BOX 6.3**

### "THE MORE WE UNDERSTAND, THE MORE WE CAN HELP"

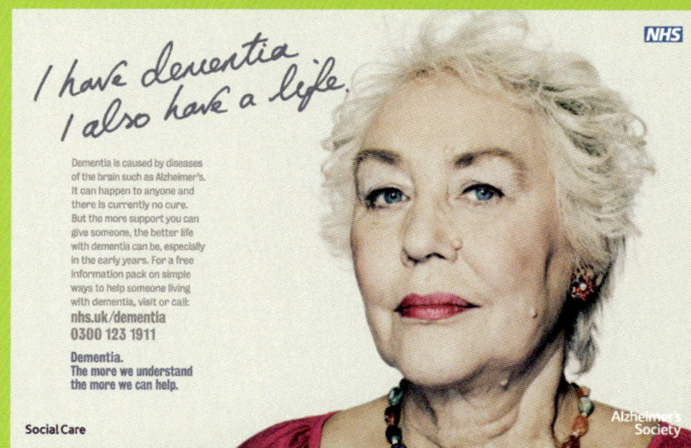
I have dementia
I also have a life.
Dementia is caused by diseases of the brain such as Alzheimer's. It can happen to anyone and there is currently no cure. But the more support you can give someone, the better life with dementia can be, especially in the early years. For a free information pack on simple ways to help someone living with dementia, visit or call:
nhs.uk/dementia
0300 123 1911
Dementia.
The more we understand the more we can help.
Social Care
NHS

Photo credit: Alzheimer's Society and the Department of Health, England.
*Source: Reference 369.*

## THEME 5: PROVIDING INFORMATION ABOUT RISK FACTORS

Factual information can be used in a number of ways to raise the level of understanding across society, including the political arena and people with dementia and their families. In some countries, campaigns that target risk reduction provide information based on best available evidence. See, for example, the Australian programme, "Mind Your Mind" (Box 6.4).

# DEVELOPING A CAMPAIGN

There are some key steps to designing a campaign. These include:

**Knowing the local context:** Collect evidence relating to the target group (regional or country prevalence data and survey results on local understanding of and attitudes to dementia). A campaign will be more successful if its messages are based on local data, and if sources of support and potential barriers to its uptake are identified.

**Involving key stakeholders:** The campaign should involve working collaboratively with the key stakeholders to identify issues that are important to them. People with dementia and their families should be involved in the design, delivery and assessment. Depending on the campaign, other stakeholders may include health professionals, school children, public servants etc.

**Determining the target audience:** The message or content will vary according to the audience. For example, the key messages will be different for people concerned about their memory, people with dementia, family members who are supporting a person with dementia, the general public, and health and social care professionals. People from different cultural backgrounds may require a different approach to meet their needs. For instance, research conducted among different minority communities highlights particular challenges in raising awareness of dementia.

**Identifying the key messages:** Messages should be clear, simple and easy to understand. Test the messages for understanding and responsiveness with a representative sample from the target audience. Campaigns should also be conducted on a long-term, routine basis to have a sustainable impact. For target groups with low literacy, pictorial and other means of conveying the information should be considered.

**Identifying the most effective way(s) to reach the target audience:** Consider the age, culture and level of literacy of the target audience. For the campaign to be effective, it should be carried out in local language/s. For example, the Alzheimer Society of Canada launched its national awareness campaign "Forget Everything You Knew" to raise public awareness and understanding of the disease in many languages. The campaign has produced television spots in Arabic, Chinese, English, French, Italian, Punjabi, Spanish and Urdu *(378)*. Depending on the target audience, print media, radio, television or web sites may be more effective. An upcoming avenue that could be explored is the use of social media for raising awareness of the younger generation.

**Being flexible in approach:** The campaign needs to evolve in response to changes in audiences, changes in the context, and changes in the social expectations of those being targeted. A good campaign is not defined only by its specific communication actions (such as the number of messages on specific channels over a specific time period) but by the methods employed for changing messages and diffusing them over time.

**Monitoring and evaluation:** Evaluation should be built into the campaign. Identify and include measurable outcomes. This will provide a benchmark for future strategies as well as providing feedback to the funding source of the benefits or otherwise of their investment to the campaign.

An improved public understanding of dementia has the capacity to improve all aspects of a person's journey through dementia. Successful awareness-raising should lead to earlier help-seeking for those who have concerns about dementia, more acceptance and greater inclusion within the community and, importantly, a more proactive community that is aware of potential risks to developing dementia.

For maximum impact, public awareness-raising should not exist in isolation. Efforts to improve awareness and knowledge within the workforce, for instance, will ease the process of help-seeking and receiving a diagnosis. Similarly, greater understanding within the political arena should result in awareness-raising being integrated into the national dementia policy, plan or strategy.

BOX 6.4

## MIND YOUR MIND, AUSTRALIA

The government-funded, Mind your Mind programme was launched by Alzheimer's Australia in 2005 to educate Australians about what they can do to reduce their risk of dementia. The programme comprises seven "signposts" to dementia risk reduction, addressing physical, mental and social activity, cardiovascular risk factors, diet, smoking and alcohol, and prevention of head injuries. It is based on epidemiological evidence of associations between dementia risk and these lifestyle and health factors, and on evidence that reducing risk factors may have significant impact on future dementia prevalence.

The Mind your Mind programme provides community education sessions, training for staff to deliver the sessions, a range of printed resources, regular promotion through the general media, an application for mobile devices, and a dedicated dementia risk-reduction web site. Materials are regularly updated as new evidence emerges.

Evaluation of the programme and of the information provided is being undertaken. Evaluation participants indicate a high level of satisfaction with their interaction with Mind your Mind, increased knowledge about dementia risk factors, and increased intention to modify their behaviour to address risk factors.

*Source: References 374–377.*

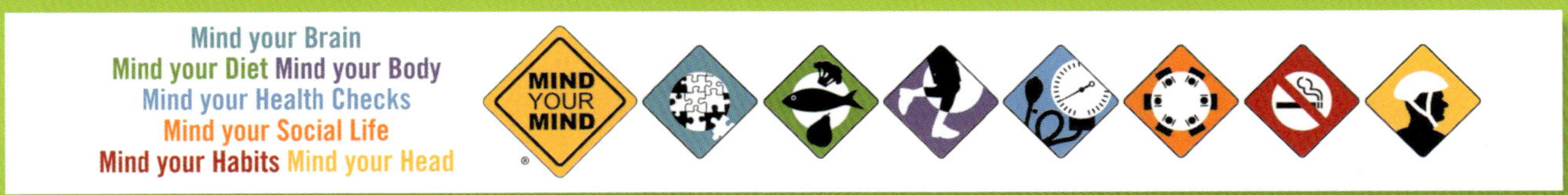
Mind your Brain
Mind your Diet Mind your Body
Mind your Health Checks
Mind your Social Life
Mind your Habits Mind your Head
MIND YOUR MIND

# RAISING AWARENESS IN THE POLITICAL SPHERE: THE ROLE OF ADVOCACY

Advocacy is crucial for making changes to policy on dementia. Its effectiveness requires the collaboration of all stakeholders: organizations for people with dementia and family organizations, medical professionals and their associations, researchers and policy-makers. The role of the media is also important for without public attention it is unlikely that the situation will change. Advocacy for dementia care should be aimed not just at health systems because other areas such as social services, employment and legal and fiscal systems are important components of policy. Alzheimer associations have been very active in their advocacy efforts in high-income countries. They have been a potent influence in raising awareness about the burden of dementia and directing public and private efforts to the development of dementia policies and plans, as in Europe and the USA (Box 6.5).

Some examples of advocacy include:

- Involvement of people with dementia as well as family caregivers, as spokespersons in their countries. Their voices and faces are powerful, especially people with a high public profile (past examples include first ladies and government ministers).

- Champions within the Department or Ministry of Health and/or Parliament who play an important role. Examples include the Alzheimer Study Group, a bipartisan body called for by leaders in the United States Congress, and the European Alzheimer's Alliance in the European Parliament.

In most LMIC advocacy is largely underdeveloped. Even so, there have been some examples from LMIC where advocacy had a role to play to bring the public's concerns about dementia to decision-makers. For example, the Alzheimer's and Related Disorders Society of India developed the *Dementia India Report* in 2010 (Box 3.4). It estimated that that the numbers of people with dementia in India was 3.7 million and that this number would double in the next 20 years. The report also provided evidence-based policy recommendations. The report facilitated the initiation of action in the country. The Government of India is discussing the establishment of the National Institute of Ageing as well as special provisions for people with dementia in the National Policy for Older People and the National Mental Health Programme during the next five-year plan *(149)*.

The challenges of developing advocacy in LMIC cannot be underestimated, but the potential benefits in terms of more appropriate resources and attention to dementia make investments in advocacy very attractive. The global advocacy community has a role to play in assisting those in LMIC with information and strategies, while respecting the local political and social structures. As is the case with other approaches for dementia care, much of this work must take place person-to-person and country-by-country.

**BOX 6.5**

## PEOPLE ADVOCATING FOR CHANGE (NATIONAL ALZHEIMER'S PROJECT ACT, USA)

In January 2011, US President Barack Obama signed into law the National Alzheimer's Project Act, which requires the government to create a National Alzheimer's Plan to address the growing dementia epidemic in the United States. Enactment of this legislation followed an extensive and widespread effort among grassroots advocates to convince the government that action was urgently needed.

While professional staff of the US Alzheimer's Association worked with members of the Congress and officials of the Obama administration on the issue, the Association also mobilized those living with Alzheimer's, caregivers, families, researchers, health care professionals and community leaders. Advocates were asked to express their support for the legislation with their members of Congress and with the Secretary of Health and Human Services (HHS). Over the course of 10 months, 50 000 emails were sent to Congress and 3 000 were sent to the HHS. In addition, Alzheimer's researchers biked across the country to recruit and mobilize advocates around the issue, collecting 112 000 petition signature. The Association used its key contact programme, known as Alzheimer's Ambassadors, to develop relationships with and to target key members of Congress. Over 1 000 meetings were held between advocates and elected officials or their staff.

This grassroots effort resulted in Congress unanimously approving the National Alzheimer's Project Act in December 2010. Advocates then made nearly 10 000 telephone calls to the White House urging President Obama to sign the legislation into law.

*Source: Reference 379.*

# SIX STAGES OF ACCEPTANCE OF DEMENTIA – A CIVIL SOCIETY PERSPECTIVE

Acceptance of dementia can be thought in terms of a six-stage model. Countries are at different stages of acceptance of dementia in various parts of the world. Different stages, with their own characteristics, are observable as awareness grows (Figure 6.1). Some countries are still at stage 1 (ignoring the problem). First

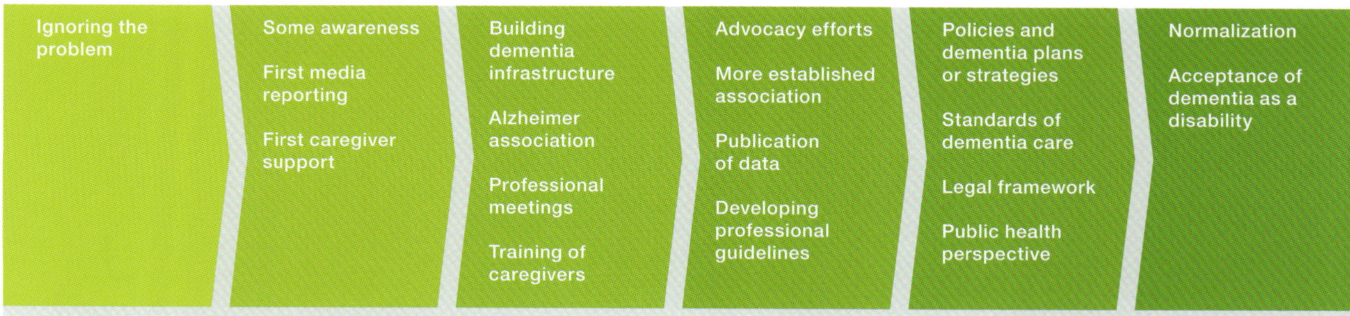


**FIG 6.1** Six stages of acceptance of dementia

steps consist of providing information by medical specialists to caregivers who are concerned about their family members (stage 2). When this reaches the media, more people become aware. The important next stage (stage 3) is building a "dementia infrastructure". This often starts with a civil society organization such as an Alzheimer association which may comprise medical and care professionals as well as family caregivers. In many countries the family caregivers are the drivers of these organizations. In some other countries it starts from a university hospital or care service facility. Their first activities may include public meetings, caregiver training, information for professionals, telephone help-lines and publications.

When the associations become more established, they recognize the need to influence the health care system (stage 4) in order to be able to extend their reach. They advocate to government and policy-makers in their country or region. This is achieved by collecting data on, for instance, prevalence and availability of services, as well as developing professional guidelines and gathering more specialized information on specific topics. Many examples exist (e.g. the *Dementia Economic Impact Report 2008* published by Alzheimers New Zealand which is used for advocacy work) *(380)*. The annual report, *Alzheimer's Disease Facts and Figures,* published by the Alzheimer's Association in the USA, is another such example. In just five years, it has become the most cited source covering the broad spectrum of dementia issues in the USA and is used frequently by policy-makers and the news media *(381)*.

Success results in progressing to stage 5, the emergence of a policy agenda, which may include the development of a dementia policy or plan by the government. A dementia policy or plan should include improved access to services, awareness-raising campaigns, better care, promotion of early diagnosis, workforce education and a research agenda (see chapter 3 for details). It may result in a stronger legal framework for the rights of people with dementia and access to financial support both for people with dementia and their caregivers. In a few countries the development of a public health perspective on dementia is seen as in Australia, England, France, Norway, the Republic of Korea and Sweden.

The sixth stage has not yet been reached anywhere and should be the culmination of these efforts: the acceptance of dementia as a disability and the inclusion of people with dementia in society as much as possible. A promising approach towards this stage is the concept of "dementia-friendly communities" which are emerging in some places *(381)*.

## SUMMARY POINTS

- Research shows that public awareness of dementia is growing, especially in high-income countries. However, public understanding is mixed and there is a fear associated with dementia which contributes to the stigma attached to the syndrome and the delay or failure in seeking help.
- There is an urgent need for improving the awareness and understanding of dementia across all levels of society in order to improve the quality of life for people with dementia and their caregivers.
- Awareness-raising and improved understanding can reduce the stigma associated with dementia and reduce the fear of the disease. Better understanding in society generally and among those who provide the care should increase help-seeking and help-giving.
- For campaigns to be effective, civil society has a role in advocating to ensure that dementia receives multi-agency government support and results in the development of sustainable, integrated programmes and supportive structures to improve the quality of life of people with dementia and their families.
- Governments have a role to play in resourcing public awareness campaigns and ensuring that key stakeholders are involved in such campaigns.
- Awareness-raising campaigns should be relevant to the context and audience, as well as effective and informative.

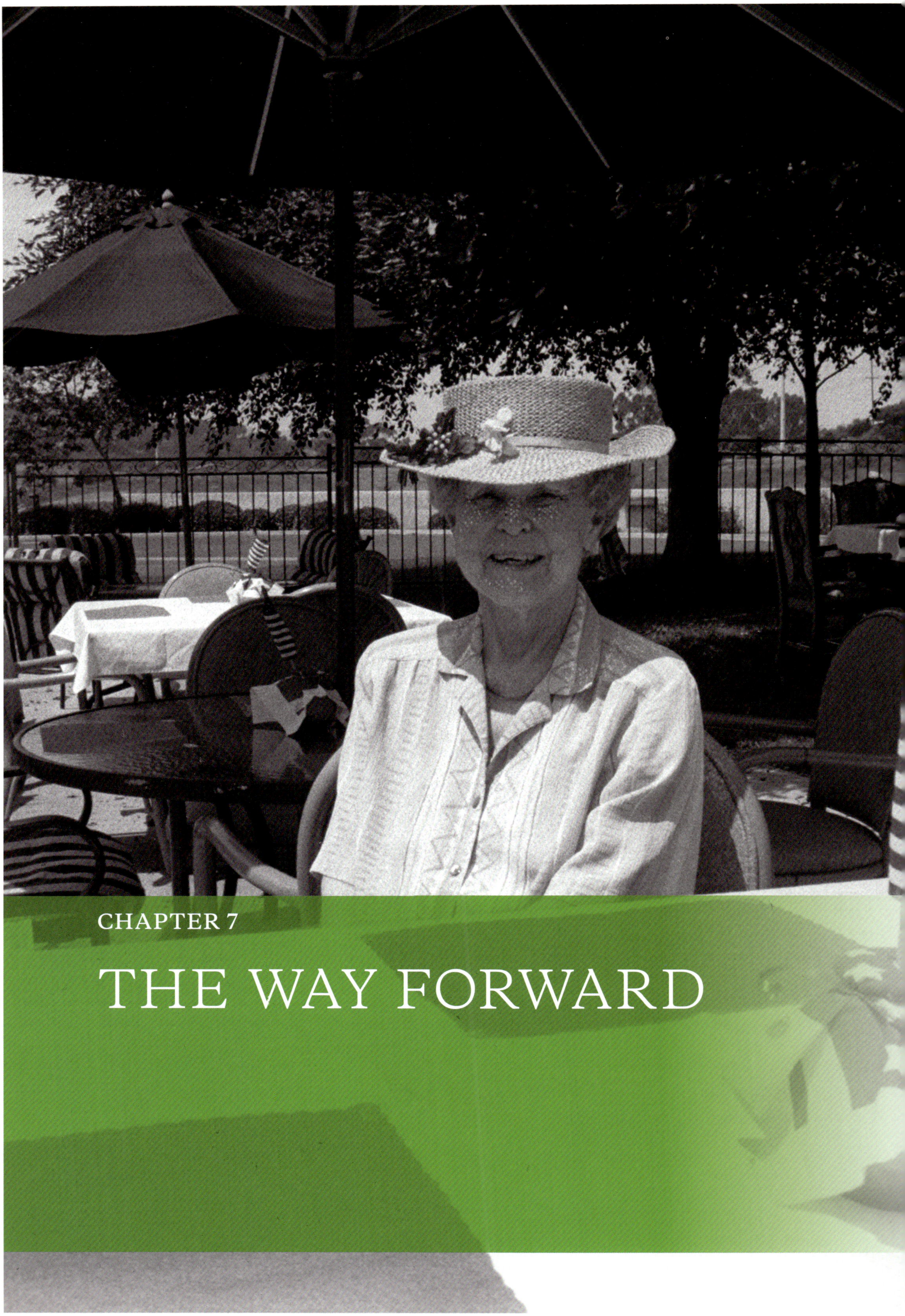

CHAPTER 7

# THE WAY FORWARD

The preceding chapters demonstrate that dementia is a global public health challenge and that urgent action is required to support country preparedness for the increasing burden and cost of dementia. This is particularly so for LMIC, which face the largest growth in numbers of persons with dementia and have limited infrastructure and health workforce capacity to address health and social problems. The findings presented in earlier chapters suggest that there is an "action gap" between knowledge of what works and concrete steps to implement it. A number of actions are thus required to improve care and services for people with dementia and their caregivers. Successful implementation of these actions will require the combined efforts of many over a sustained period.

This chapter summarizes the need for action. It describes a framework for undertaking action, delineating the areas in which this is required and the roles of the different stakeholders.

## THE NEED FOR ACTION

There is little doubt that dementia poses one of the greatest societal challenges for the 21st century that must be addressed internationally, nationally and locally, as well as at family and personal levels. Dementia is exceptional in terms of size, cost and impact. Our world had 35.6 million people with dementia in 2010 – 0.5% of the world's population – and this number is projected to double every 20 years to over 115 million in 2050. Currently, 58% of people with dementia live in LMIC, and this proportion is projected to increase to 71% by 2050.

The costs of dementia are estimated at US$ 604 billion per year at present and are rising more quickly than prevalence of the condition. The impact of dementia on socioeconomic conditions worldwide is enormous. Furthermore, dementia is highly stigmatized and universally feared, with studies suggesting that it is strongly associated with suffering, disability and economic loss at all stages of a person's journey through dementia *(365)*.

It is important to address the question of what action has been taken so far and, if it is relatively little, why that might be. Barriers to prioritization include the complexity of dementia care which involves health and social care, the family, and the private and voluntary sectors. This obscures recognition of who should take responsibility, complicates financing, and therefore hinders the process of advocacy and action. There are also powerful societal misconceptions concerning dementia – that it is not a very common problem, that it is a normal part of ageing, that there is nothing that can be done to help, that it is better not to know, and that it is the families' responsibility to provide care. These misconceptions, which are the norm rather than the exception, reinforce beliefs that dementia is not an issue for health care systems or governments. They are shared by many politicians, policy-makers, health administrators and health professionals. They are generally benignly held but they result in a lack of prioritization of dementia and therefore a lack of action.

The direct result is that, worldwide, the large majority of people with dementia and their family caregivers do not benefit from the positive intervention and support that can promote independence and maintain quality of life. Timely diagnosis and early intervention can help people with dementia and their families to steer a course through the 7–12 years that they may be living with dementia, and will assist them to avoid crises and promote their well-being *(179)*. Unfortunately, as identified in chapter 4, data from high-income countries reveal that only one fifth to one half of cases of dementia are recognized and documented in primary care case note records *(179)*. The National Audit Office, reviewing the United Kingdom system, concluded that only about a third of people with dementia receive a diagnosis of dementia. When they receive that diagnosis, it is usually late in the disorder, often at a time of crisis when it is too late to prevent the harm that has been caused both to the person with dementia and the family *(144)*. Many current systems require fundamental redesign of services.

Political commitment is needed to generate strategies, policies, programmes and services that work for people with dementia. Strategies and their implementation can be at the level of health services, or at sub-national level, but coordinating and direction is also required nationally and internationally in view of the global nature of the coming epidemic and its profound fiscal and societal impacts.

# THE VALUE OF ACTION

At the launch of the five-year French national plan in February 2008, President Nicolas Sarkozy of France expressed an urgent need for change *(383)*:

... When the suffering of a loved one affects a whole family, I know we can wait no longer and that every day counts. Today I am launching a five-year National Plan for Alzheimer's. This is a lasting State commitment in the battle that we wage against the disease. It is also a personal commitment from me.

As chapter 3 outlined, there are initiatives in progress in countries and in diverse systems, though primarily in high-income countries. These initiatives vary but generally include a mixture of high-level (often five-year) strategic planning for quality improvement in dementia care, with specific clinical, social and research commitments. Their scope is comprehensive and their intention is to provide the policy framework for local service development. These documents are therefore not only political statements but guidance for developing and commissioning health and social services that meet the needs of those affected.

The value of the action that has been identified by countries can be viewed from three main perspectives, namely:

- the value of alleviating suffering;
- the value of strategic management of cost;
- the social value of intervention.

**The value of alleviating suffering:** This is an altruistic motive that acknowledges first the profound impact of dementia on the quality of life of those affected and of their families. It also accepts that interventions that are clinically- and cost-effective should be made available.

When launching England's national dementia strategy, Alan Johnson, the Secretary of State for Health, stated that:

"Dementia is not an illness we can ignore. It has a devastating impact on the people who develop it, and the families who care for them ... That is why the government has made dementia a national priority ..."

**The value of the strategic management of cost:** The societal cost of dementia is high, but it may be possible to "invest to save". Effective dementia care may cost less in the long term than ineffective and inefficient provision. The main cost driver in all systems is the cost of long-term care, particularly when provided in care homes. Such care is expensive, often of low quality, and dreaded by many of those who may need to use it. There is a win-win-win situation generated by early effective clinical intervention, by improving quality of life, by preventing long-term harm and by decreasing cost *(179, 384)*. A national consensus may be required for the foresight needed to embrace a 5–10-year reward horizon after initial investment.

**The social value of intervention:** Societies worldwide are undergoing profound and rapid change. Established cultural norms of care and social protection provided by extended family networks are no longer sustainable and will become less so over time. Planning for the long-term care of people with dementia is therefore a key policy priority. This requires a national debate regarding the needs for long-term care, eligibility, financing and the respective roles of family and state.

# THE FRAMEWORK FOR ACTION

The effective implementation of efforts to address the global burden of dementia requires that certain actions be executed and that they involve researchers, practitioners, civil society organizations, policy-makers, health planners and international development agencies. The key actions include advocacy and awareness-raising, developing and implementing dementia policies and plans, health system strengthening, capacity-building, supporting caregivers and research. These actions need to be context-specific and culturally relevant. All of them require financial, technical and human resources.

## ADVOCACY AND AWARENESS-RAISING

Advocacy for policy change and awareness-raising are two distinct actions. Both approaches are critical and are complementary to each other. The first targets governments at local, national and international levels with the aim of encouraging policies that will improve dementia care and services. The second focuses on people with dementia, their families and society in general, aiming to improve their understanding of dementia and to change public attitudes and practices. This in turn creates a demand for services and builds capacity for grass-roots advocacy and for holding governments to account. Even in the absence of an ideal policy environment, well-constructed population-level awareness-raising efforts can help people with dementia and their families to be in a stronger and better-informed position to seek a diagnosis, plan for the future, and make more appropriate use of health and social services. Advocacy efforts in high-income countries have grown with increasing intensity over the past decades, with some initiatives also from LMIC. Civil society organizations such as Alzheimer associations have spearheaded this push (see chapter 6). The task of convincing government financers, development assistance agencies and other donors that investment in dementia care and services is critical is a challenging one, especially in view of constrained budgets and many competing health and development priorities. Media advocacy, social marketing and social mobilization can serve as conduits of information and as mechanisms for advocacy to build support among the various global health and development stakeholders.

Both in coordination with policy changes and as a separate action for overcoming the stigma surrounding dementia, there is substantial promise in implementing awareness-raising efforts. Public communication efforts that are coordinated with policy changes can enhance the effectiveness of both approaches and, together, can help create an environment in which more targeted programmes in health and social care systems and communities can succeed. Depending on the infrastructure within a country, efforts to raise awareness can occur at multiple levels, from the national government to local authorities and community-based organizations.

## DEVELOPING AND IMPLEMENTING DEMENTIA POLICIES AND PLANS

A coordinated multisectoral approach is required for comprehensive policy development, involving relevant government departments, civil society and the private sector. National action is essential for systems change to become a reality. The issues and actions related to dementia could be part of a separate strategy, policy or plan or included in general health, ageing or mental health policy, depending upon the country's context.

The policies and plans will remain on paper unless implementation issues are addressed. A broad-based set of programmatic initiatives will need to be implemented in a sustained fashion in order to improve dementia care and services. These programmes should include a range of approaches such as awareness-raising, risk reduction, early diagnosis and treatment, continuing and integrated care through the health and social care sectors, financial and legal protection, workforce education, and research. Financial commitment is required for optimal implementation of dementia policies and plans. Depending on the existing infrastructure, national and subnational authorities are responsible for implementing public health and health and social care programmes. Other programme implementers include universities, NGOs and other organizations in civil society and, in some LMIC, development agencies.

## HEALTH AND SOCIAL SYSTEMS STRENGTHENING

There is widespread acceptance that only through building or strengthening health and social systems will outcomes for people with dementia and their caregivers be improved. To achieve the goals, it is essential that health and social services are equipped to provide the range of care and services required for persons with dementia and their caregivers. The capacity of health and social workers needs to be built so that they work in ways that are responsive, fair and efficient to achieve the best health outcomes possible with the resources available. Investment in health information systems is needed in order to develop, improve and standardize methods for collection of data on the health determinants and health status of people with dementia and their caregivers. In addition, a good health financing system is required to ensure that people with dementia and their caregivers can use needed services and are protected from financial catastrophe or impoverishment if they have to pay for them.

For resource-poor settings, such as in many LMIC, WHO's Mental Health Gap Action Programme (mhGAP) *(181)* has explicitly acknowledged the need for building health systems. An important component of the programme is capacity-building and task-shifting (i.e. from specialists to the much more numerous nonspecialist health and social care professionals) if coverage of effective care is to be extended to all who need it. Task-sharing may be a more appropriate term, since specialists have an essential role in all health systems, whether in planning services or in training, supporting and supervising those who deliver care at the primary care level. Thus capacity-building is necessary at all levels of the health and social care systems, providing relevant knowledge and skills to nonspecialists and increasing the number and variety of specialists to support them. The role of caregivers as important service providers – together with their needs for information, education and skills training – must not be forgotten. It will require years of sustained support and investment to meet gaps in capacity needs in LMIC and to have a meaningful impact. Engaging academia, NGOs and government institutions, as well as training government health officials in the effective use of relevant policies and the effective management and maintenance of programmes, is crucial.

The dominant global health agenda is undergoing a paradigm shift, marked by the recent United Nations high-level meeting on noncommunicable disease prevention and control *(8)*. Strengthening the health systems and the workforce to prevent, treat and control major chronic diseases provides opportunities and threats – opportunities because chronic disease care paradigms apply equally to dementia care as to diabetes, and threats because dementia, the most costly and disabling of all chronic disease conditions, is not prioritized in the newly emerging consensus for action. Nevertheless, the impetus for international action resulting from the high-level meeting and its focus on noncommunicable diseases presents an unprecedented opportunity to raise the priority of dementia worldwide.

## RESEARCH AND EVALUATION

Research evidence should underpin all actions and is a critical element of the overall package of global dementia efforts. Each country should determine a priority research agenda. There is also need for international collaboration and private/public sector partnerships to address important shared concerns such as the development of new and more effective treatments. In general, more should be invested in projects that generate knowledge about how to translate what is already known into action and implementation – in other words, to close the knowledge – action gap. This agenda will be multidisciplinary, spanning basic sciences, health services, health systems and health policy research. Countries need to monitor the course of the dementia epidemic for changes in prevalence and incidence that might indicate the success or failure of measures taken to control it, and for uptake of services to assess progress towards closing the treatment gap. Significantly more research is needed to better understand the causes of dementia and how and when lifestyle factors influence the risk for developing it; such knowledge can inform effective prevention strategies. A balance must be struck between research into treatment, care and cure on the one hand and pharmacological and psychosocial intervention approaches on the other.

To date, most research has been carried out in high-income countries. As well as adapting what is known to work in high-income countries and applying it to LMIC realities, there may be opportunities to draw on health system and service innovation from resource-poor LMIC in order to increase the efficiency and effectiveness of care in all settings.

## KEY MESSAGES

- Dementia is not a normal part of ageing.
- 35.6 million people were estimated to be living with dementia in 2010. There are 7.7 million new cases of dementia each year, implying that there is a new case of dementia somewhere in the world every four seconds. The accelerating rates of dementia are cause for immediate action, especially in LMIC where resources are few.
- The huge cost of the disease will challenge health systems to deal with the predicted future increase of prevalence. The costs are estimated at US$ 604 billion per year at present and are set to increase even more quickly than the prevalence.
- People live for many years after the onset of symptoms of dementia. With appropriate support, many can and should be enabled to continue to engage and contribute within society and have a good quality of life.
- Dementia is overwhelming for the caregivers and adequate support is required for them from the health, social, financial and legal systems.
- Countries must include dementia on their public health agendas. Sustained action and coordination is required across multiple levels and with all stakeholders – at international, national, regional and local levels.
- People with dementia and their caregivers often have unique insights to their condition and life. They should be involved in formulating the policies, plans, laws and services that relate to them.
- The time to act is now by:
  - promoting a dementia friendly society globally;
  - making dementia a national public health and social care priority worldwide;
  - improving public and professional attitudes to, and understanding of, dementia;
  - investing in health and social systems to improve care and services for people with dementia and their caregivers;
  - increasing the priority given to dementia in the public health research agenda.

# REFERENCES


1. Presidential Proclamation – National Alzheimer's Disease Awareness Month, 2011. Washington, DC, The White House, 2011 (http://www.aaacap.org/The%20 White%20House_National%20Alzheimer's%20Disease%20Awareness%20Month, %202011_Proclamation.htm accessed 8 December 2011).
2. International statistical classification of diseases and related health problems, 10th Revision. Geneva, World Health Organization, 1992.
3. World Alzheimer's Report 2009. London, Alzheimer's Disease International, 2009.
4. Neurological disorders: public health challenges. Geneva, World Health Organization, 2006.
5. World Population Ageing 2009. New York, NY, United Nations, 2009 (http://www.un.org/esa/population/publications/WPA2009/WPA2009_WorkingPaper.pdf accessed 4 February 2012).
6. The global burden of disease: 2004 update. Geneva, World Health Organization, 2008.
7. World Alzheimer's Report 2010: the global economic impact of dementia. London, Alzheimer's Disease International, 2010.
8. Political Declaration of the High-level Meeting of the General Assembly on the Prevention and Control of Non-communicable Diseases, 19-20 September 2011. New York, NY, United Nations, 2011 (Document A/66/L.1; http://www.un.org/ga/search/view_doc.asp?symbol=A/66/L.1, accessed 4 February 2012).
9. mhGAP Intervention Guide for mental, neurological and substance use disorders in non-specialized health settings. Geneva, World Health Organization, 2010.
10. mhGAP Evidence Resource Centre. Geneva, World Health Organization (online portal to WHO mental health resources at http://www.who.int/mental_health/mhgap/evidence/en/index.html, accessed 4 February 2012).
11. World population prospects: the 2002 revision – highlights. New York, United Nations, 2003.
12. Ferri CP et al. Global prevalence of dementia: a Delphi consensus study. Lancet, 2005, 366 (9503): 2112–2117.
13. Herrera E Jr et al. Epidemiologic survey of dementia in a community-dwelling Brazilian population. Alzheimer Disease & Associated Disorders, 2002, 16 (2): 103–108.
14. Nitrini R et al. Incidence of dementia in a community-dwelling Brazilian population. Alzheimer Disease & Associated Disorders, 2004, 18 (4): 241–246.
15. Rosselli D et al. The Mini-Mental State Examination as a selected diagnostic test for dementia: a Colombian population study. Revista De Neurologia, 2000, 30 (5): 428–432.
16. Hendrie HC et al. Prevalence of Alzheimer's disease and dementia in two communities: Nigerian Africans and African Americans. American Journal of Psychiatry, 1995, 152: 1485–1492.
17. The 10/66 Dementia Research Group. Methodological issues in population-based research into dementia in developing countries. A position paper from the 10/66 Dementia Research Group. International Journal of Geriatric Psychiatry, 2000, 15: 21–30.
18. Chandra V et al. Prevalence of Alzheimer's disease and other dementias in rural India. The Indo-US study. Neurology, 1998, 51: 1000–1008.
19. Canadian Study of Health and Ageing. Canadian study of health and aging: study methods and prevalence of dementia. Canadian Medical Association Journal, 1994, 5, 150 (6): 899–913.
20. Llibre Rodriguez JJ et al. Prevalence of dementia in Latin America, India, and China: a population-based cross-sectional survey. Lancet, 2008, 372 (9637): 464–474.
21. Llibre RJ et al. The prevalence, correlates and impact of dementia in Cuba. A 10/66 group population-based survey. Neuroepidemiology, 2008, 31 (4): 243–251.
22. Farrag A et al. Prevalence of Alzheimer's disease and other dementing disorders: Assiut-Upper Egypt study. Dementia and Geriatric Cognitive Disorders, 1998, 9 (6): 323–928.
23. Reynish E et al. EUROCODE: Report of WP7 2006. Prevalence of dementia in Europe. Alzheimer Europe, 2006 (http://ec.europa.eu/health/archive/ph_information/dissemination/diseases/docs/eurocode.pdf, accessed 4 February 2012).
24. Kokmen E et al. Prevalence of medically diagnosed dementia in a defined United States population: Rochester, Minnesota, January 1, 1975. Neurology, 1989, 39 (6): 773–776.
25. Ott A et al. Prevalence of Alzheimer's disease and vascular dementia: association with education. The Rotterdam study. British Medical Journal, 1995, 310 (6985): 970–973.
26. Knapp M, Prince M. Dementia UK – A report into the prevalence and cost of dementia prepared by the Personal Social Services Research Unit (PSSRU) at the London School of Economics and the Institute of Psychiatry at King's College London, for Alzheimer's Society. London, Alzheimer's Society, 2007.
27. Ratnavalli E et al. The prevalence of frontotemporal dementia. Neurology, 2002, 58 (11): 1615–1621.
28. Harvey RJ, Skelton-Robinson M, Rossor MN. The prevalence and causes of dementia in people under the age of 65 years. Journal of Neurology, Neurosurgery and Psychiatry, 2003, 74 (9): 1206–1209.
29. Shaji S et al. An epidemiological study of dementia in a rural community in Kerala, India. British Journal of Psychiatry, 1996, 168 (6): 745–749.
30 Vas CJ et al. Prevalence of dementia in an urban Indian population. International Psychogeriatrics/IPA, 2001, 13 (4): 439–450.
31. McArthur JC et al. Human immunodeficiency virus-associated neurocognitive disorders: Mind the gap. Annals of Neurology, 2010, 67 (6): 699–714.
32. Sacktor N. The epidemiology of human immunodeficiency virus-associated neurological disease in the era of highly active antiretroviral therapy. Journal of Neurovirology, 2002, 8 (Suppl 2): 115–121.
33. Joska JA et al. Characterization of HIV-associated neurocognitive disorders among individuals starting antiretroviral therapy in South Africa. AIDS and Behaviour, 2011, 15 (6): 1197–1203.
34. Prince M et al. No health without mental health. Lancet, 2007, 370 (9590): 859–877.
35. Dong MJ et al. The prevalence of dementia in the People's Republic of China: a systematic analysis of 1980–2004 studies. Age and Ageing, 2007, 36 (6): 619–264.
36. Hofman A et al. The prevalence of dementia in Europe: a collaborative study of 1980–1990 findings. Eurodem Prevalence Research Group. International Journal of Epidemiology, 1991, 20 (3): 736–748.
37. Lobo A et al. Prevalence of dementia and major subtypes in Europe: a collaborative study of population-based cohorts. Neurologic Diseases in the Elderly Research Group. Neurology, 2000, 54 (11, Suppl 5): S4–S9.
38. Guerchet M, et al. Cognitive impairment and dementia in elderly people living in rural Benin, West Africa. Dementia and Geriatric Cognitive Disorders, 2009; 27 (1): 34–41.
39. Guerchet M et al. Prevalence of dementia in elderly living in two cities of Central Africa: the EDAC survey. Dementia and Geriatric Cognitive Disorders, 2010, 30 (3): 261–268.
40. Paraiso MN et al. Prevalence of dementia among elderly people living in Cotonou, an urban area of Benin (West Africa). Neuroepidemiology, 2011, 36 (4): 245–251.
41. Yusuf AJ et al. Prevalence of dementia and dementia subtypes among community-dwelling elderly people in northern Nigeria. International Psychogeriatrics/IPA, 2011, 23 (3): 379–386.
42. Prince M et al. Dementia diagnosis in developing countries: a cross-cultural validation study. Lancet, 2003, 361 (9361): 909–917.
43. Prince M et al. The 10/66 Dementia Research Group's fully operationalised DSM IV dementia computerized diagnostic algorithm, compared with the 10/66 dementia algorithm and a clinician diagnosis: a population validation study. BMC Public Health, 2008, 8: 219 (doi: 10.1186/1471-2458-8-219).
44. Jotheeswaran AT, Williams JD, Prince MJ. The predictive validity of the 10/66 dementia diagnosis in Chennai, India: a 3-year follow-up study of cases identified at baseline. Alzheimer Disease and Associated Disorders, 2010, 24 (3): 296–302.
45. Neuropathology Group of the Medical Research Council Cognitive Function and Aging Study. Pathological correlates of late-onset dementia in a multicentre, community-based population in England and Wales. Neuropathology Group of the Medical Research Council Cognitive Function and Ageing Study (MRC CFAS). Lancet, 2001 357 (9251): 169–175.
46. Jellinger KA. Clinicopathological analysis of dementia disorders in the elderly – an update. Journal of Alzheimer's Disease, 2006, 9 (3 Suppl): 61–70.
47. Snowdon DA et al. Brain infarction and the clinical expression of Alzheimer disease. The Nun Study. Journal of the American Medical Association, 1997, 277 (10): 813–817.
48. O'Connor DW et al. The prevalence of dementia as measured by the Cambridge Mental Disorders of the Elderly Examination. Acta Psychiatrica Scandinavica, 1989, 79 (2): 190–198.
49. Brayne C, Calloway P. An epidemiological study of dementia in a rural population of elderly women. British Journal of Psychiatry, 1989, 155: 214–219.
50. Clarke M et al. The prevalence of dementia in a total population: a comparison of two screening instruments. Age and Ageing, 1991, 20 (6): 396–403.

51. Stevens T et al. Islington study of dementia subtypes in the community. British Journal of Psychiatry, 2002, 180: 270–276.

52. McGonigal G et al. Epidemiology of Alzheimer's presenile dementia in Scotland, 1974–88. British Medical Journal, 1993, 306 (6879): 680–683.

53. Newens AJ et al. Clinically diagnosed presenile dementia of the Alzheimer type in the Northern Health Region: ascertainment, prevalence, incidence and survival. Psychological Medicine, 1993, 23 (3): 631–644.

54. Suh GH, Shah A. A review of the epidemiological transition in dementia-cross-national comparisons of the indices related to Alzheimer's disease and vascular dementia. Acta Psychiatrica Scandinavica, 2001, 104 (1): 4–11.

55. Ziegler-Graham K et al. Worldwide variation in the doubling time of Alzheimer's disease incidence rates. Alzheimer's and Dementia, 2008, 4 (5): 316–323.

56. Jorm AF, Jolley D. The incidence of dementia: a meta-analysis. Neurology, 1998, 51 (3): 728–733.

57. Fitzpatrick AL et al. Survival following dementia onset: Alzheimer's disease and vascular dementia. Journal of the Neurological Sciences, 2005, 229–230: 43–49.

58. Hendrie HC et al. Incidence of dementia and Alzheimer disease in 2 communities: Yoruba residing in Ibadan, Nigeria, and African Americans residing in Indianapolis, Indiana.. Journal of the American Medical Association, 2001, 285 (6): 739–747.

59. Chandra V et al. Incidence of Alzheimer's disease in a rural community in India: the Indo-US study. Neurology, 2001, 57 (6): 985–989.

60. Hendrie HC et al. Alzheimer's disease, genes, and environment: the value of international studies. Canadian Journal of Psychiatry, 2004 49 (2): 92–99.

61. Deeg M et al. A comparison of cardiovascular disease risk factor biomarkers in African Americans and Yoruba Nigerians. Ethnicity and Disease, 2008, 18 (4): 427–433.

62. Dewey ME, Saz P. Dementia, cognitive impairment and mortality in persons aged 65 and over living in the community: a systematic review of the literature. International Journal of Geriatric Psychiatry, 2001, 16 (8): 751–761.

63. Perkins AJ et al. Risk of mortality for dementia in a developing country: the Yoruba in Nigeria. International Journal of Geriatric Psychiatry, 2002, 17 (6): 566–573.

64. Nitrini R et al. Mortality from dementia in a community-dwelling Brazilian population. International Journal of Geriatric Psychiatry, 2005, 20 (3): 247–253.

65. Jotheeswaran AT, Williams JD, Prince MJ. Predictors of mortality among elderly people living in a south Indian urban community; a 10/66 Dementia Research Group prospective population-based cohort study. BMC Public Health, 2010, 10: 366.

66. Access Economics PTY Limited. The dementia epidemic: economic impact and positive solutions for Australia. Canberra, Access Economics PTY Limited, 2003.

67. Rising tide: the impact of dementia on Canadian society. A study commissioned by the Alzheimer Society. Toronto, Alzheimer Society of Canada, 2010.

68. Wimo A, Johansson L, Jönsson L. Demenssjukdomarnas samhällskostnader och antalet dementa i Sverige 2005 (The societal costs of dementia and the number of demented in Sweden 2005) (in Swedish). Stockholm, Socialstyrelsen, 2007 (Report No.: 2007-123-32).

69. US Alzheimer's Association. 2010 Alzheimer's disease facts and figures. Alzheimer's and Dementia, 2010, 6 (2): 158–194.

70. Wimo A et al. The economic impact of dementia in Europe in 2008 – cost estimates from the Eurocode project. International Journal of Geriatric Psychiatry, 2011, 26 (8): 825-832.

71. Wang H et al. Caregiver time and cost of home care for Alzheimer's disease: a clinic-based observational study in Beijing, China. Ageing International, 2010, 35 (2): 153-165.

72. Wang G et al. Economic impact of dementia in developing countries: an evaluation of Alzheimer-type dementia in Shanghai, China. Journal of Alzheimer's Disease, 2008, 15 (1): 109–115.

73. Allegri RF et al. Economic impact of dementia in developing countries: an evaluation of costs of Alzheimer-type dementia in Argentina. International Psychogeriatrics/IPA, 2007, 19 (4): 705–718.

74. Zencir M et al. Cost of Alzheimer's disease in a developing country setting. International Journal of Geriatric Psychiatry, 2005, 20 (7): 616–622.

75. Williams A. Calculating the global burden of disease: time for a strategic reappraisal? Health Economics, 1999, 8 (1): 1–8.

76. Wimo A, Jonsson L, Winblad B. An estimate of the worldwide prevalence and direct costs of dementia in 2003. Dementia and Geriatric Cognitive Disorders, 2006, 21 (3): 175–181.

77. Wimo A, Winblad B, Jonsson L. An estimate of the total worldwide societal costs of dementia in 2005. Alzheimer's and Dementia, 2007, 3 (2): 81–91.

78. Wimo A, Winblad B, Jonsson L. The worldwide societal costs of dementia: Estimates for 2009. Alzheimers and Dementia, 2010, 6 (2): 98–103.

79. Wimo A, Prince M. World Alzheimer Report 2010; the global economic impact of dementia. London, Alzheimer's Disease International, 2010.

80. Macdonald A, Cooper B. Long-term care and dementia services: an impending crisis. Age and Ageing, 2007, 36 (1): 16–22.

81. Luengo-Fernandez R, Leal J, Gray A. Dementia 2010. The prevalence, economic cost and research funding of dementia compared with other major diseases. A report produced by the Health Economics Research Centre, University of Oxford for the Alzheimer's Research Trust. Cambridge, Alzheimer's Research Trust, 2010.

82. Wimo A, Johansson L, Jonsson L. [Prevalence study of societal costs for dementia 2000–2005. More demented people – but somewhat reduced costs per person] (in Swedish). Lakartidningen, 2009, 106 (18–19): 1277–1282.

83. Daviglus ML et al. Risk factors and preventive interventions for Alzheimer disease: state of the science. Archives of Neurology, 2011, 68 (9): 1185–1190.

84. Hofman A et al. Atherosclerosis, apolipoprotein E, and prevalence of dementia and Alzheimer's disease in the Rotterdam Study. Lancet, 1997, 349: 151–154.

85. Ott A et al. Smoking and risk of dementia and Alzheimer's disease in a population-based cohort study: the Rotterdam Study. Lancet, 1998, 351: 1841–1843.

86. Juan D et al. A 2-year follow-up study of cigarette smoking and risk of dementia. European Journal of Neurology, 2004, 11 (4): 277–282.

87. Luchsinger JA et al. Aggregation of vascular risk factors and risk of incident Alzheimer disease. Neurology, 2005, 65 (4): 545–551.

88. Tyas SL et al. Mid-life smoking and late-life dementia: the Honolulu-Asia Aging Study. Neurobiology of Aging, 2003, 24 (4): 589–596.

89. Whitmer RA et al. Midlife cardiovascular risk factors and risk of dementia in late life. Neurology, 2005, 64 (2): 277–281.

90. Ott A et al. Diabetes mellitus and the risk of dementia: the Rotterdam Study. Neurology, 1999, 53 (9): 1937–1942.

91. Skoog I et al. 15-year longitudinal study of blood pressure and dementia. Lancet, 1996, 347 (9009): 1141–1145.

92. Kivipelto M et al. Midlife vascular risk factors and Alzheimer's disease in later life: longitudinal, population based study. British Medical Journal, 2001, 322 (7300): 1447–1451.

93. Yip AG, Brayne C, Matthews FE. Risk factors for incident dementia in England and Wales: The Medical Research Council Cognitive Function and Ageing Study. A population-based nested case-control study. Age and Ageing, 2006, 35 (2): 154–160.

94. Bursi F et al. Heart disease and dementia: a population-based study. American Journal of Epidemiology, 2006, 163 (2): 135–141.

95. Casserly I, Topol E. Convergence of atherosclerosis and Alzheimer's disease: inflammation, cholesterol, and misfolded proteins. Lancet, 2004, 363 (9415): 1139–1146.

96. Stewart R et al. Twenty-six-year change in total cholesterol levels and incident dementia: the Honolulu-Asia Aging Study. Archives of Neurology, 2007, 64 (1): 103–107.

97. Stewart R et al. A 32-year prospective study of change in body weight and incident dementia: the Honolulu-Asia Aging Study. Archives of Neurology, 2005, 62 (1): 55–60.

98. McGuinness B et al. Statins for the prevention of dementia. The Cochrane Database of Systematic Reviews, 2009, (2): CD003160.

99. McGuinness B, Todd S, Passmore P, Bullock R. The effects of blood pressure lowering on development of cognitive impairment and dementia in patients without apparent prior cerebrovascular disease. The Cochrane Database of Systematic Reviews, 2006, (2): CD004034.

100. Valenzuela MJ, Sachdev P. Brain reserve and dementia: a systematic review. Psychological Medicine, 2006, 36 (4): 441–454.

101. Li G et al. A three-year follow-up study of age-related dementia in an urban area of Beijing. Acta Psychiatrica Scandinavica, 1991, 83 (2): 99–104.

102. Barnes DE, Whitmer RA, Yaffe K. Physical activity and dementia: the need for prevention trials. Exercise and Sport Sciences Reviews, 2007, 35 (1): 24–29.

103. Ahlskog JE et al. Physical exercise as a preventive or disease-modifying treatment of dementia and brain aging. Mayo Clinic Proceedings, 2011, 86 (9): 876–884.

104. Angevaren M et al. Physical activity and enhanced fitness to improve cognitive function in older people without known cognitive impairment. The Cochrane Database of Systematic Reviews, 2008, (3): CD005381.

105. Barnes DE, Yaffe K. The projected effect of risk factor reduction on Alzheimer's disease prevalence. Lancet Neurology, 2011, 10 (9): 819–828.

106. Epping-Jordan JE et al. Preventing chronic diseases: taking stepwise action. Lancet, 2005, 366 (9497): 1667–1671.

107. Plassman BL et al. Prevalence of dementia in the United States: the aging, demographics, and memory study. Neuroepidemiology, 2007, 29 (1–2): 125–132.

108. Gurvit H et al. The prevalence of dementia in an urban Turkish population. American Journal of Alzheimer's Disease and Other Dementias, 2008, 23 (1): 67–76.

109. Hendrie HC et al. Incidence of dementia and Alzheimer disease in 2 communities: Yoruba residing in Ibadan, Nigeria, and African Americans residing in Indianapolis, Indiana. Journal of the American Medical Association, 2001, 285 (6): 739–747.

110. Chandra V et al. Incidence of Alzheimer's disease in a rural community in India: the Indo-US study. Neurology, 2001, 57 (6): 985–989.

111. Prince M et al. The protocols for the 10/66 Dementia Research Group population-based research programme. BMC Public Health, 2007, 7 (1): 165.

112. Dunn G et al. Two-phase epidemiological surveys in psychiatric research. British Journal of Psychiatry, 1999, 174: 95–100.

113. Prince M. Commentary: two-phase surveys. A death is announced; no flowers please. International Journal of Epidemiology, 2003, 32 (6): 1078–1080.

114. Sousa RM et al. The contribution of chronic diseases to the prevalence of dependence among older people in Latin America, China and India: a 10/66 Dementia Research Group population-based survey. BMC Geriatrics, 2010, 10 (1): 53.

115. Rocca WA et al. Frequency and distribution of Alzheimer's disease in Europe: a collaborative study of 1980-1990 prevalence findings. The EURODEM-Prevalence Research Group. Annals of Neurology, 1991, 30 (3): 381–390.

116. Prince MJ et al. The 10/66 Dementia Research Group's fully operationalised DSM-IV dementia computerized diagnostic algorithm, compared with the 10/66 dementia algorithm and a clinician diagnosis: a population validation study. BMC Public Health, 2008, 8: 219.

117. Ganguli M et al. Classification of neurocognitive disorders in DSM-5: a work in progress. American Journal of Geriatric Psychiatry, 2011, 19 (3): 205–210.

118. International Advisory Group for the Revision of ICD-10 Mental and Behavioural Disorders. A conceptual framework for the revision of the ICD-10 classification of mental and behavioural disorders. World Psychiatry, 2011, 10: 86-92.

119. Dias A, Patel V. Closing the treatment gap for dementia in India. Indian Journal of Psychiatry, 2009, 51 (5): 93–97.

120. Everybody's business: strengthening health systems to improve health outcomes. Geneva, World Health Organization, 2007.

121. Living well with dementia: A National Dementia Strategy. Leeds, Department of Health, 2009 (http://www.dh.gov.uk/prod_consum_dh/groups/dh_digitalassets/@dh/@en/documents/digitalasset/dh_094051.pdf, accessed 4 February 2012).

122. Dementia initiative national evaluation: overview and summary of main findings. Final report. Report of the LAMA Consortium. Canberra, Department of Health and Ageing, 2009 (http://www.health.gov.au/internet/main/publishing.nsf/Content/500DD5C951D7E214CA2578170017A8F9/$File/LAMAOverview.pdf, accessed 4 February 2012).

123. Ontario's Strategy for Alzheimer Disease and Related Dementias: PREPARING FOR OUR FUTURE. Toronto, Ministry of Health and Long-Term Care, 1999 (http://www.health.gov.on.ca/english/public/pub/ministry_reports/alz/alz_strat.pdf, accessed 4 February 2012).

124. National Handlingsplan For Demensindsatsen. (National dementia plan available in Danish). Copenhagen, Ministry of Social Affairs and Integration, 2010 (http://www.sm.dk/Data/Dokumentertilpublikationer/Publikationer%202010/Demensindsats%202010/Demens_handlingsplan14-12.pdf, accessed 4 February 2012).

125. French National Plan for "Alzheimer and related diseases" 2008–2012. Paris, Ministry of Health, 2008 (http://www.plan-alzheimer.gouv.fr/IMG/pdf/A_short_summary_of_Plan_Alzheimer_2008-2012_as_of_30_june_2011.pdf).

126. Emergency project for improvement of medical care and quality of life for people with dementia. Project report. (In Japanese). Tokyo, Ministry of Health, Labour and Welfare, 2008 (http://www.mhlw.go.jp/houdou/2008/07/dl/h0710-1a.pdf, accessed 4 February 2012).

127. Takeda A, Tanaka N, Chiba T. Prospects of future measures for persons with dementia in Japan. Psychogeriatrics, 2010, 10 (2): 95–101.

128. Lee S. Commentary: Dementia strategy Korea. International Journal of Geriatric Psychiatry, 2010, 25 (9): 931-932.

129. National strategies to address dementia. Scullin, Alzheimer's Australia, 2011 (http://www.fightdementia.org.au/common/files/NAT/20111410_Paper_25_low_v2.pdf, accessed 4 February 2012).

130. Caring for people with dementia. Statement by the President of the Dutch House of Representatives. The Hague, Ministry of Health, Welfare and Sport, 2008 (http://english.minvws.nl/en/kamerstukken/lz/2009/caring-for-people-with-dementia.asp, accessed 4 February 2012).

131. Improving Dementia Services in Northern Ireland. Department of Health, Social Services and Public Safety, 2011 (http://www.dhsspsni.gov.uk/improving-dementia-services-in-northern-ireland-a-regional-strategy-november-2011.pdf, accessed 4 February 2012).

132. Dementia plan 2015. Oslo, Norwegian Ministry of Health and Care Services, 2007 (http://www.regjeringen.no/upload/HOD/Dokumenter%20KTA/DementiaPlan2015.pdf, accessed 4 February 2012).

133. Scotland's National Dementia Strategy. Edinburgh, The Scottish Government, 2010. (http://www.scotland.gov.uk/Resource/Doc/324377/0104420.pdf, accessed 20 January 2012).

134. Maladie d'Alzheimer et maladies apparentées. Lausanne, Canton of Vaud, 2010 (http://www.vd.ch/fileadmin/user_upload/themes/sante_social/services_soins/Sant%C3%A9_mentale/fichier_pdf/Synth%C3%A8se___Programme_Alzheimer.29.11.2010.pdf, accessed 4 February 2012).

135. Alzheimer's Associations. State Government Alzheimer's Disease Plans. (http://www.alz.org/join_the_cause_state_plans.asp, accessed 4 February 2012).

136. National dementia vision for Wales. Cardiff, Welsh Assembly Government, 2011 http://wales.gov.uk/docs/dhss/publications/110302dementiaen.pdf, accessed 4 February 2012).

137. Burns A. Editorial. International Journal of Geriatric Psychiatry, 2010, 25 (9): 875.

138. Alzheimer Europe. National dementia plans. (http://www.alzheimer-europe.org/Policy-in-Practice2/National-Dementia-Plans, accessed 9 December 2011).

139. Eriksson S. Developments in dementia strategy. International Journal of Geriatric Psychiatry, 2010, 25 (9): 885–886.

140. National guidelines for care in cases of dementia. Stockholm, National Board of Health and Welfare (Socialstyrelsen), 2010 (http://www.socialstyrelsen.se/nationalguidelines/nationalguidelinesforcareincasesofdementia, accessed 12 February 2012).

141. Kyoto Declaration: Minimum actions required for the care of people with dementia. 20th International Conference of Alzheimer's Disease International, Kyoto, Japan. Kyoto, Alzheimer's Disease International, 2004 (http://www.alz.co.uk/adi/pdf/kyotodeclaration.pdf, accessed 12 February 2012).

142. World health report 2001. Geneva, World Health Organization, 2001.

143. Paris Declaration. Paris, Alzheimer Europe, 2006 (http://www.alzheimer-europe.org/EN/Policy-in-Practice2/Paris-Declaration, accessed 12 February 2012).

144. Improving services and support for people with dementia. London, National Audit Office, 2007 (http://www.nao.org.uk/publications/0607/dementia_services_and_support.aspx, accessed 12 February 2012).

145. Public Accounts Committee. Improving services and support for people with dementia. London, The Stationery Office, 2008 (http://www.publications.parliament.uk/pa/cm200708/cmselect/cmpubacc/228/228.pdf, accessed 12 February 2012).

146. Services for older adults. Center for Studies on Aging (http://csa.org.lb/en/default.asp?menuID=4, accessed 4 February 2012).

147. Mental health atlas 2011. Geneva, World Health Organization, 2011.

148. Uwakwe R et al. The epidemiology of dependence in older people in Nigeria: prevalence, determinants, informal care, and health service utilization. A 10/66 Dementia Research Group cross-sectional survey. Journal of the American Geriatrics Society, 2009, 57 (9): 1620–1627.

149. The Dementia India Report 2010: prevalence, impact, costs and services for dementia. New Delhi, Alzheimer's and Related Disorders Society of India, 2010 (http://www.alzheimer.org.in/dementia_2010.pdf, accessed 5 February 2011).

150. Closing the gap in a generation: health equity through action on the social determinants of health. Final report of the Commission on Social Determinants of Health. Geneva, World Health Organization, 2008.

151. Population ageing and development – new strategies for social protection. Report of a seminar held on 31 October 2002 at the National Press Club, Washington, DC, USA. London, HelpAge International, 2003 (www.helpage.org/download/4c4627dfabf3a/, accessed 12 February 2012).

152. Heavy reliance on out of pocket expenditures leads to financial barriers for poor. WHO/NHA Policy Highlight No.2/May 2011. Geneva, World Health Organization, 2011 (http://www.who.int/nha/use/2008data_highlight2.pdf, accessed 12 February 2012).

153. Acosta et al. The epidemiology of dependency among urban-dwelling older people in the Dominican Republic; a cross-sectional survey. BMC Public Health, 2008, 8: 285.

154. Centre for Health Statistics and Information, Ministry of Health. An analysis report of national health services survey in 2003. Beijing, Chinese Academy Science & Peking Union Medical College, 2004.

155. Liu Z et al. Chronic disease prevalence and care among the elderly in urban and rural Beijing, China – a 10/66 Dementia Research Group cross-sectional survey . BMC Public Health, 2009, 9: 394.

156. Wagstaff A et al. Extending health insurance to the rural population: an impact evaluation of China new cooperative scheme. Journal of Health Economics, 2009, 28 (1): 1–19.

157. Prince M et al. Alzheimer Disease International's 10/66 Dementia Research Group – one model for action research in developing countries. International Journal of Geriatric Psychiatry, 2004, 19 (2): 178–181.

158. Prince M. The 10/66 dementia research group – 10 years on. Indian Journal of Psychiatry, 2009, 51 (Suppl 1): S8–S15.

159. Garcez-Leme L E, Leme MD, Espino DV. Geriatrics in Brazil: a big country with big opportunities. Journal of the American Geriatrics Society, 2005, 53: 2018–2022.

160. Non-contributory pensions and poverty prevention. A comparative study of Brazil and South Africa. Final report. London, Institute of Development and Policy Management, 2003.

161. World health report 2010. Health systems financing: the path to universal coverage. Geneva, World Health Organization, 2010.

162. Matsuda S, Yamamoto M. Long-term care insurance and integrated care for the aged in Japan. International Journal of Integrated Care, 2001, 1: e28.

163. Convention on the Rights of Persons with Disabilities. New York, NY, United Nations, 2006 (http://www.un.org/disabilities/convention/conventionfull.shtml, accessed 4 February 2012).

164. Centre for Disability Law and Policy. Submission on Legal Capacity to Oireachtas Committee on Justice, Defence and Equality, 2011 (http://www.nuigalway.ie/cdlp/documents/cdlp_submission_on_legal_capacity_the_oireachtas_committee_on_justice_defence_and_equality_.pdf, accessed 12 February 2012).

165. Capezuti E. Minimizing the use of restrictive devices in dementia patients at risk for falling. Nursing Clinics of North America, 2004, 39 (3): 625–647.

166. Wang W-W, Moyle W. Physical restraint use on people with dementia: A review of the literature. Australian Journal of Advanced Nursing, 2005, 22 (4): 46–52.

167. Comparative analysis of legislation in Europe relating to the rights of people with dementia. Final report. Luxembourg, Alzheimer Europe, 2005.

168. Dementia: ethical issues. London, The Nuffield Council on Bioethics, 2009 (http://www.nuffieldbioethics.org/go/ourwork/dementia/publication_530.html, accessed 4 February 2012).

169. Nidus Personal Planning Resource Centre and Registry (British Columbia, Canada) (http://www.nidus.ca/, accessed 8 December 2011).

170. Sweden Personal Ombudsman Model (http://www.po-skane.org/, accessed 8 December 2011).

171. Powers BA. Nursing home ethics: everyday issues affecting residents with dementia. New York, Springer, 2001.

172. Baldwin C et al. Making difficult decisions: the experience of caring for someone with dementia. London, Alzheimer's Society, 2005.

173. Hughes J, Baldwin C. Ethical issues in dementia care: making difficult decisions. London, Jessica Kingsley, 2006.

174. Lindemann H. Care in families. In: Ascroft RE et al., eds. Principles of health care ethics, 2nd edition. Chichester, John Wiley & Sons, 2007.

175. Bamford C et al. Disclosing a diagnosis of dementia: a systematic review. International Journal of Geriatric Psychiatry, 2004, 19: 151–169.

176. Fisk JD et al. Disclosure of the diagnosis of dementia. Alzheimer's and Dementia, 2007, 3 (4): 404–410.

177. Abma TA, Molewijk AC, Widdershoven GAM. Good care in ongoing dialogue: Improving the quality of care through moral deliberation and responsive evaluation. Health Care Analysis, 2009, 17 (3): 217–235.

178. van der Dam S et al. "Here's my dilemma". Moral case deliberation as a platform for discussing everyday ethics in elderly care. Health Care Analysis, 2011, DOI: 10.1007/s10728-011-0185-9.

179. World Alzheimer's Report 2011: the benefits of early diagnosis and intervention. London, Alzheimer's Disease International, 2011.

180. Dias A, Patel V. Closing the treatment gap for dementia in India. Indian Journal of Psychiatry, 2009, 51 (5): 93–97.

181. mhGAP: Mental Health Gap Action Programme: scaling up care for mental, neurological, and substance use disorders. Geneva, World Health Organization, 2008.

182. Dementia across Australia: 2011-2050. Deloitte Access Economics, 2011 (http://www.fightdementia.org.au/common/files/NAT/20111014_Nat_Access_DemAcrossAust.pdf, accessed 12 February 2012).

183. Brodaty H, Cumming A. Dementia services in Australia. International Journal of Geriatric Psychiatry, 2010, 25: 887–895.

184. Wimo A et al. Patients with dementia in group living: experiences 4 years after admission. International Psychogeriatrics/IPA, 1995, 7 (1): 123–127.

185. Mejia-Arango S, Gutierrez LM. Prevalence and incidence rates of dementia and cognitive impairment no dementia in the Mexican population: data from the Mexican health and aging study. Journal of Aging and Health, 2011, 23: 1050–1074.

186. Pinquart M, Sorensen S. Helping caregivers of persons with dementia: which interventions work and how large are their effects? International Psychogeriatrics/IPA, 2006, 18: 577–595.

187. Lee H, Cameron ML. Respite care for people with dementia and their carers (Review). The Cochrane Library, 2008, Issue 3.

188. Auer SR et al. A 10 day training program for persons with dementia and their carers: a practical nonpharmacological treatment program. Alzheimer's and Dementia, 2009, 5 (4) (Suppl1): 406.

189. Auer S et al. Entlastung pflegender Angehöriger: Ein Programm der M.A.S Alzheimerhilfe. Zeitschrift für Gerontopsychologie & -psychiatrie, 2007, 20 (2/3): 169–174.

190. Kitwood T. Cultures of care: tradition and change. In: Benson S, Kitwood T (eds.) The new culture of dementia care. London, Hawker, 1995.

191. Kitwood T. Dementia reconsidered: the person comes first. Buckingham, Open University Press, 1997.

192. Chenoweth L et al. Caring for Aged Dementia Care Resident Study (CADRES) of person-centred care, dementia-care mapping, and usual care in dementia: a cluster-randomised trial. Lancet Neurology, 2009; published online 12 March.

193. WHO definition of palliative care. Geneva, World Health Organization, 2002 (http://www.who.int/cancer/palliative/definition/en, accessed 5 February 2012).

194. Small N, Downs M, Froggatt K. Improving end of life care for people with dementia: The benefits of combining UK approaches to palliative care and dementia care. In: Miesen BML, Jones GMM (eds.) Care giving in dementia: research and applications. Vol. 4. London, Routledge, 2006.

195. Hughes JC et al. Palliative care in dementia: issues and evidence. Advances in Psychiatric Treatment, 2007, 13: 251–260.

196. Holmervova I et al. Dignity and palliative care in dementia. Journal of Nutrition, Health and Ageing, 2007, 11 (6): 489–494.

197. Organisation for Economic Cooperation and Development. Ensuring quality long-term care for older people. OECD Observer Policy Brief, March 2005 (http://www.oecd.org/dataoecd/53/4/34585571.pdf, accessed 5 February 2012).

198. Organisation for Economic Cooperation and Development (OECD). Help Wanted? Providing and Paying for Long-Term Care. OECD Publishing, 2011 (http://www.oecd.org/document/23/0, 3746, en_2649_37407_47659479_1_1_1_37407, 00.html#TOC, accessed 14 February 2012).

199. From red to gray. The "third transition" of ageing populations in Eastern Europe and the Former Soviet Union. Washington, DC, The World Bank, 2007.

200. Nikmat AW, Hawthorne G, Hassan Ahmad Al-Mashoor S. Dementia In Malaysia: issues and challenges. ASEAN Journal of Psychiatry, 2011, 12 (1): Jan–June 2011.

201. Prince MJ et al. Packages of care for dementia in low and middle income countries. PLoS Medicine, 2009, 6e 1000176.

202. Smith K et al. High prevalence of dementia and cognitive impairment in Indigenous Australians. Neurology, 2008, 71 (19): 1470–1473.

203. Alzheimer's Australia. Dementia: a major health problem for indigenous people. Briefing prepared for Parliamentary Friends of Dementia. Paper No. 12, August 2007 (http://www.fightdementia.org.au/common/files/NAT/20070800_Nat_NP_12DemMajHlthProblndig.pdf, accessed 6 February 2012).

204. Beattie A et al. "They don't quite fit the way we organize our services" – Results from a UK field study of marginalized groups and dementia care. Disability and Society, 2005, 20 (1): 67–80.

205. Bowes A, Wilkinson H. "We didn't know it would get that bad": South Asian experiences of dementia and the service response. Health and Social Care in the Community, 2003, 11 (5): 387–397.

206. Mukadam N, Cooper C, Livingston G. A systematic review of ethnicity and pathways to care in dementia. International Journal of Geriatric Psychiatry, 2011, 26: 12–20.

207. Low LF et al. Recognition, attitudes and causal beliefs regarding dementia in Italian, Greek and Chinese Australians. Dementia and Geriatric Cognitive Disorders, 2010, 30 (6): 499–508.

208. Venessa Curnow, National Aboriginal & Torres Strait Islander Liaison Officer & Director, National Congress of Australia's First Peoples. (Personal communication).

209. Arkles R et al. Ageing, cognition and dementia in Australian aboriginal and Torres Strait Islander Peoples: a life cycle approach. Neuroscience Research Australia and Muru Marri Indigenous Health Unit, University of New South Wales, 2010 (http://www.neura.edu.au/sites/neura.edu.au/files/Full%20Literature%20Review%20Aug2010.pdf, accessed 10 February 2012).

210. Beginning the conversation: addressing dementia in Aboriginal and Torres Strait Islander communities. Canberra, Alzheimer's Australia, 2006 (http://www.fightdementia.org.au/understanding-dementia/aboriginal-and-torres-strait-islander-resources-and-publications.aspx, accessed 7 November 2011).

211. National Task Group on Intellectual Disabilities and Dementia Practice. "My thinker's not working": a national strategy for enabling adults with intellectual disabilities affected by dementia to remain in their community and receive quality supports. The American Academy of Developmental Medicine and Dentistry, the Rehabilitation Research and Training Center on Aging with Developmental Disabilities-Lifespan Health and Function at the University of Illinois at Chicago, and the American Association on Intellectual and Developmental Disabilities, 2012. (http://aadmd.org/sites/default/files/NTG_Thinker_Report.pdf, accessed 10 February 2012).

212. Downs M et al. Caring for patients with dementia: the GP perspective. Aging and Mental Health, 2000, 4 (4): 301–304.

213. Downs M. The role of general practice and the primary care team in dementia diagnosis and management. International Journal of Geriatric Psychiatry, 1996, 11: 937–942.

214. Turner S et al. General practitioners' knowledge, confidence and attitudes in the diagnosis and management of dementia. Age and Ageing, 2004, 33: 461–467.

215. Iliffe S, Wilcock J. The identification of barriers to the recognition of, and response to, dementia in primary care using a modified focus group approach. Dementia, 2005, 4 (1): 73–85.

216. Koch T, Iliffe S. Rapid appraisal of barriers to the diagnosis and management of patients with dementia in primary care: a systematic review. BMC Family Practice, 2010, 11 (52): 1–8.

217. De Lepeleire JA et al. How do general practitioners diagnose dementia? Family Practice, 1994, 11 (2): 148–152.

218. Cahill S et al. The attitudes and practices of general practitioners regarding dementia diagnosis in Ireland. International Journal of Geriatric Psychiatry, 2008, 23: 663–669.

219. Iliffe S, Manthorpe J, Eden A. Sooner or later? Issues in the early diagnosis of dementia in general practice: a qualitative study. Family Practice, 2003, 20 (4): 376–381.

220. Vernooij-Dassen M J et al. Factors affecting timely recognition and diagnosis of dementia across Europe: from awareness to stigma. International Journal of Geriatric Psychiatry, 2005, 20: 377–386.

221. Kaduszkiewicz H, Wiese B, Van den Bussche H. Self-reported competence, attitude and approach of physicians towards patients with dementia in ambulatory care: results of a postal survey. BMC Health Services Research, 2008, 8 (54): 1–10.

222. Brodaty H et al. General practice and dementia. The Medical Journal of Australia, 1994, 160 (1): 10–14.

223. Iliffe S et al. Understanding obstacles to the recognition of and response to dementia in different European countries: a modified focus group approach using multinational, multi-disciplinary expert groups. Aging and Mental Health, 2005, 9 (1): 1–6.

224. Prepared to care: challenging the dementia skills gap. London, All-Party Parliamentary Group on Dementia, 2009.

225. Public awareness of dementia: what every commissioner needs to know. London, Alzheimer's Society, 2009.

226. Dementia. London, United Kingdom Department of Health (http://www.dh.gov.uk/health/category/policy-areas/social-care/dementia/, accessed 8 December 2011).

227. The world health report – working together for health. Geneva, World Health Organization, 2006 (http://www.who.int/whr/2006/en/index.html, accessed 26 November 2011).

228. Alfonso T, Krishnamoorthy ES, Gomez K. Caregiving for dementia: global perspectives and transcultural issues. In: Krishnamoorthy ES, Prince MJ, Cummings JL, eds. Dementia: a global approach. Cambridge, Cambridge University Press, 2010.

229. Otero et al. Regional dementia networks: a step towards integrated community dementia care. In preparation.

230. Krishnamoorthy ES, Gilliam F. Best clinical and research practice in adult epileptology. Epilepsy & Behavior, 2009, 15 (Suppl. 1): S55-59.

231. Gould E, Reed P. Alzheimer's Association quality care campaign and professional training initiatives: improving hands-on care for people with dementia in the USA. International Psychogeriatics/IPA, 2009, 21: 25–33.

232. Teri L et al. Staff training in assisted living: evaluating treatment fidelity. International Journal of Geriatric Psychiatry, 2010, 18: 502–509.

233. Babu Varghese, Project Officer, The Alzheimer's and Related Disorders Society of India. (Personal communication).

234. Testad I et al. Nursing home structure and association with agitation and use of psychotropic drugs in nursing home residents in three countries: Norway, Austria and England. International Journal of Geriatric Psychiatry, 2009, 25 (7): 725-731.

235. Dias A et al. The effectiveness of a home care programme for supporting caregivers of persons with dementia in developing countries: a randomized controlled trial from Goa, India. PLoS ONE, 2008, 4 June, 3 (6): e2333.

236. Gavrilova SI et al. Helping carers to care. The 10/66 dementia research group's randomized control trial of a caregiver intervention in Russia. International Journal of Geriatric Psychiatry, 2009, 24: 347–354.

237. Guerra M et al. Helping carers to care: the 10/66 dementia research group's randomized control trial of a caregiver intervention in Peru. Revista brasileira de psiquiatria (Brazilian Journal of Psychiatry), 2010 (2 July), pii: S1516-4446201 0005000017.

238. Dementia: a NICE-SCIE guideline on supporting people with dementia and their carers in health and social care. National clinical practice guideline No. 42. London, British Psychological Society and Gaskell, 2007.

239. Management of patients with dementia. A national clinical guideline. Edinburgh, Scottish Intercollegiate Guidelines Network (SIGN), 2006 (SIGN publication No. 86).

240. Wind A et al. NHG-Standarad dementie (tweede herziening) [Dutch College of General Practitioners Dementia guideline]. Huisarts en Wetenschap, 2003, 46 (13): 754–767.

241. National Guideline Clearinghouse. (http://www.guideline.gov/, accessed 12 February 2012).

242. Allegri RF et al. Enfermedad de Alzheimer. Guía de práctica clínica. Neurología Argentina, 2011, 3: 2: 120–137.

243. Diagnostico y ratamiento de las Demencia en el Adulto Mayor en el Primer Nivel de Atención. Mexico City, Instituto Mexicano del Seguro Social, 2010 (http://www.imss.gob.mx/SiteCollectionDocuments/migracion/profesionales/GuiasClinicas/DEMENCIA_AM_EVR_CENETEC_13092010.pdf, accessed 5 February 2012).

244. Diagnóstico y Tratamiento de la Demencia Vascular. Mexico City, Secretaria de Salud, 2011 (http://www.cenetec.salud.gob.mx/descargas/gpc/CatalogoMaestro/450_GPC_Demencia_vascular/GER_Demencia_vascular.pdf, accessed 5 February 2012).

245. Quality Dementia Care Series (1–6). Canberra, Alzheimer's Australia, 2003–2009. (http://www.fightdementia.org.au/research-publications/quality-dementia-care-papers.aspx, accessed 6 February 2012).

246. Barbui C et al. Challenges in developing evidence-based recommendations using the GRADE approach: the case of mental, neurological, and substance use disorders. PLoS Medicine, 2010, 31 August, 7 (8).

247. Dua T et al. Evidence-based guidelines for mental, neurological, and substance use disorders in low- and middle-income countries: Summary of WHO recommendations. PLoS Medicine, 2011, 15 November, 8 (11): e1001122.

248. Common core principles for supporting people with dementia: a guide to training the social care and health workforce. Leeds, Skills for Care & Skills for Health, 2011 (http://www.dh.gov.uk/prod_consum_dh/groups/dh_digitalassets/documents/digitalasset/dh_127587.pdf, accessed 5 February 2012).

249. Banerjee, S. The use of anti-psychotic medications for people with dementia. A report for the Minister of State for Care Services (http://www.nhs.uk/news/2009/10October/Pages/Antipsychotic-use-in-dementia.aspx, accessed 5 February 2012).

250. Lustenberger I et al. Psychotropic medication use in Swiss nursing homes. Swiss Medical Weekly, 2011, 141: w13254.

251. Gauthier S et al. Management of behavioral problems in Alzheimer's disease. International Psychogeriatrics/IPA, 2010, 22 (3): 346–372 (Epub 2010 Jan 25).

252. Antipsychotic drugs for dementia: a balancing act. Lancet Neurology, 2009, 8: 125.

253. Conventional and atypical antipsychotics and antidepressant (trazodone) for behavioural and psychological symptoms in people with dementia. mhGAP evidence resource centre (http://www.who.int/mental_health/mhgap/evidence/dementia/q3/en/index.html, accessed 5 February 2012).

254. Doyle M, Timmonen V. The different faces of care work: understanding the experiences of the multi-cultural care workforce. Ageing and Society, 2009, 29: 337–350.

255. Howe AL. Migrant careworkers or migrants working in long term care? Journal of Ageing and Social Policy, 2009 21: 374–392.

256. Mears J. Global labour markets: care work and "chains of caring". Thesis. Sydney, University of Western Sydney.

257. Success for unique dementia training course. Edinburgh, Alzheimer Scotland, 2011 (http://dementiascotland.org/news/2011/success-unique-dementia-training-course/, accessed 6 December 2011).

258. Sousa RM et al. Contribution of chronic diseases to disability in elderly people in countries with low and middle incomes: a 10/66 Dementia Research Group population-based survey. Lancet, 2009, 374 (9704): 1821–1830.

259. Schulz R, Martire LM. Family caregiving of persons with dementia: prevalence, health effects, and support strategies. The American Journal of Geriatric Psychiatry: official journal of the American Association for Geriatric Psychiatry, 2004, 12: 240–249.

260. Gaugler JE et al. (2003). Caregiving and institutionalization of cognitively impaired older people: utilizing dynamic predictors of change. Gerontologist, 43, 219–229.

261. Manton KG, Corder LS, Stallard E. Estimates of change in chronic disability and institutional incidence and prevalence rates in the US elderly population from the 1982, 1984, and 1989 National Long Term Care Survey. Journal of Gerontology, 1993, 48: S153–166.

262. Fried LP, Guralnik JM. Disability in older adults: evidence regarding significance, etiology, and risk. Journal of the American Geriatrics Society, 1997, 45: 92–100.

263. Arno PS, Levine C, Memmott MM. The economic value of informal caregiving. Health Affairs, 1999, 18: 182–188.

264. Covinsky KE et al. Reduced employment in caregivers of frail elders: impact of ethnicity, patient clinical characteristics, and caregiver characteristics. The Journals of Gerontology. Series A, Biological sciences and medical sciences, 2001, 56: 707–713.

265. Services for supporting family carers of elderly people in Europe: characteristics, coverage and usage. Summary of main findings from EUROFAMCARE. Hamburg, EUROFAMCARE, 2006 (http://www.uke.de/extern/eurofamcare/documents/deliverables/summary_of_findings.pdf, accessed 29 November 2011).

266. Disability, ageing and carers, Australia: summary of findings, 2003. Canberra, Australian Bureau of Statistics, 2004 (Cat. No. 4430) (http://www.abs.gov.au/AUSSTATS/abs@.nsf/Lookup/4430.0Main+Features12003?OpenDocument, accessed 20 January 2010).

267. Schneider J et al. EUROCARE: a cross-national study of co-resident spouse carers for people with Alzheimer's disease: I-Factors associated with carer burden. International Journal of Geriatric Psychiatry, 1999, 14 (8): 651–661.

268. Prince M. 10/66 Dementia Research Group (2004). Care arrangements for people with dementia in developing countries. International Journal of Geriatric Psychiatry, 2004, 19 (2): 170–177.

269. Kaneda T. Health care challenges for developing countries with aging populations. Washington, DC, Population Reference Bureau, 2011 (http://www.prb.org/Articles/2006/HealthCareChallengesforDevelopingCountrieswithAgingPopulations.aspx, accessed 5 December 2011).

270. Uwakwe R, Modebe I. Community and family care responses for patients with dementia in eastern Nigeria. Global Ageing, 2007, 4: 35–43.

271. 10/66 Dementia Research Group. Behavioral and psychological symptoms of dementia in developing countries. International Psychogeriatrics/IPA, 2004, 16 (4): 441–459.

272. Reisberg B. Diagnostic criteria in dementia: a comparison of current criteria, research challenges, and implications for DSM-V. Journal of Geriatric Psychiatry and Neurology, 2006, 19 (3): 137–146.

273. Neurological disorders: public health challenges. Geneva, World Health Organization, 2006.

274. Wolff JL et al. End-of-life care: findings from a national survey of informal caregivers. Archives of Internal Medicine, 2007, 167: 40–46.

275. Whitlatch CJ, Feinberg LF. Family care and decision making. In: Cox CB, ed. Dementia and social work practice: research and interventions. New York, NY, Springer Publishing Company, 2007.

276. Quinn C, Clare L, Woods RT. The impact of motivations and meanings on the wellbeing of caregivers of people with dementia: a systematic review. International Psychogeriatrics, 2010, 22: 43–55.

277. Bacon E et al. Positive experiences in caregivers: an exploratory case series. Behavioural and Cognitive Psychotherapy, 2009, 37: 94–114.

278. Uwakwe R, Modebe I. Disability and care giving in old age in a Nigerian community. Nigerian Journal of Clinical Practice, 2007, 10: 58–65.

279. Uwakwe R. Satisfaction with dementia care-giving in Nigeria: a pilot investigation. International Journal of Geriatric Psychiatry, 2006, 21: 1–2.

280. Shaji KS et al. Caregivers of people with Alzheimer's disease: a qualitative study from the Indian 10/66 Dementia Research Network. International Journal of Geriatric Psychiatry, 2003, 18 (1): 1–6.

281. O'Brien J, Ames D, Burns A. Dementia. London, Arnold, 2000.

282. Pinquart M, Sörensen S. Differences between caregivers and noncaregivers in psychological health and physical health: a meta-analysis. Psychology and Aging, 2003, 18: 250–267.

283. Pinquart M, Sorensen S. Helping caregivers of persons with dementia. Which interventions works and how large are their effects? International Psychogeriatrics, 2006, 8: 577–595.

284. Vitaliano, PP, Zhang J, Scanlan JM. Is caregiving hazardous to one's physical health? A meta-analysis. Psychological Bulletin, 2003, 129: 946–972.

285. Schulz R, Beach SR. Caregiving as a risk factor for mortality: the Caregiver Health Effects Study. Journal of the American Medical Association, 1999, 282: 2215–2219.

286. Brodaty H, Luscombe G. Psychological morbidity in caregivers is associated with depression in patients with dementia. Alzheimer Disease and Associated Disorders, 1998, 12: 62–70.

287. Cuijpers P. Depressive disorders in caregivers of dementia patients: a systematic review. Aging and Mental Health, 2005, 9: 325–330.

288. Akkerman RL, Ostwald SK. Reducing anxiety in Alzheimer's disease family caregivers: the effectiveness of a nine-week cognitive-behavioral intervention. American Journal of Alzheimer's Disease and Other Dementias, 2004, 19: 117–123.

289. Ballard CG et al. A follow up study of depression in the carers of dementia sufferers. British Medical Journal, 1996, 312: 947.

290. Miller B, Cafasso L. Gender differences in caregiving: fact or artifact? Gerontologist, 1992, 32: 498–507.

291. Yee JL, Schulz R. Gender differences in psychiatric morbidity among family caregivers: a review and analysis. Gerontologist, 2000, 40: 147–164.

292. Robinson-Whelen S et al. Long-term caregiving: what happens when it ends? Journal of Abnormal Psychology, 2001, 110: 573–584.

293. Vitaliano PP et al. Psychophysiological mediators of caregiver stress and differential cognitive decline. Psychology and Aging, 2005, 20: 402–411.

294. Vitaliano PP, Young HM, Zhang J. Is caregiving a risk factor for illness? Current Directions in Psychological Science, 2004, 13: 13–16.

295. Schulz R et al. Health effects of caregiving. The Caregiver Health Effects Study: an ancillary study of The Cardiovascular Health Study. Annals of Behavioral Medicine, 1997. 19: 110–116.

296. Kiecolt-Glaser JK et al. Spousal caregivers of dementia victims: longitudinal changes in immunity and health. Psychosomatic Medicine, 1991, 53: 345–362.

297. Kiecolt-Glaser J et al. Chronic stress alters the immune response to influenza virus vaccine in older adults. Proceedings of the Nationall Academy of Sciences of the USA, 1996, 93: 3043–3047.

298. Glaser R, Kiecolt-Glaser JK. Chronic stress modulates the virusspecific immune response to latent herpes simplex virus Type 1. Annals of Behavioral Medicine, 1997, 19: 78–82.

299. King AC, Oka RK, Young DR. Ambulatory blood pressure and heart rate responses to the stress of work and caregiving in older women. The Journals of Gerontology. Series A, Biological sciences and medical sciences, 1994, 49: 239–245.

300. Kiecolt-Glaser JK et al. Slowing of wound healing by psychological stress. Lancet, 1995, 346: 194–196.

301. Shaw WS et al. Longitudinal analysis of multiple indicators of health decline among spousal caregivers. Annals of Behavioral Medicine, 1997, 19: 101–109.

302. Alzheimer's Association. Alzheimer's disease facts and figures. Alzheimer's and Dementia: the journal of the Alzheimer's Association, 2011, 7: 208-244.

303. Smits CH et al. Effects of combined intervention programmes for people with dementia living at home and their caregivers: a systematic review. International Journal of Geriatric Psychiatry, 2007, 22: 1181–1193.

304. Brodaty H, Green A, Koschera A. Meta-analysis of psychosocial interventions for caregivers of people with dementia. Journal of the American Geriatric Society, 2003, 51: 657–664.

305. Lee H, Cameron M. Respite care for people with dementia and their carers. The Cochrane Database of Systematic Reviews, 2004: CD004396.

306. Spijker A et al. Effectiveness of nonpharmacological interventions in delaying the institutionalization of patients with dementia: a meta-analysis. Journal of the American Geriatrics Society, 2008, 56 (6): 1116–1128.

307. Olazaran J et al. Nonpharmacological therapies in Alzheimer's disease: a systematic review of efficacy. Dementia and Geriatric Cognitive Disorders, 2010, 30: 161–178.

308. Mittelman M et al. An intervention that delays institutionalization of Alzheimer's disease patients: treatment of spouse-caregivers. The Gerontologist, 1993, 33: 730–740.

309. Mittelman M et al. A family intervention to delay nursing home placement of patients with Alzheimer disease: a randomized control trial. Journal of the American Medical Association, 1996, 276: 1725–1731.

310. Mittelman M et al. Improving caregiver well-being delays nursing home placement of patients with Alzheimer disease. Neurology, 2006, 67: 1592–1599.

311. Mittelman M et al. Preserving health of Alzheimer caregivers: impact of a spouse caregiver intervention. American Journal of Geriatric Psychiatry, 2007, 15: 780–789.

312. Mittelman M et al. A 3 country randomized controlled trial of psychosocial intervention for caregivers combined with pharmacological treatment for patients with Alzheimer's disease: effects on caregiver depression. American Journal of Geriatric Psychiatry, 2008, 16: 893–904.

313. Ostwald S et al. Reducing caregiver burden: a randomized psychoeducational intervention for caregivers of persons with dementia. The Gerontologist, 1999, 39: 299–309.

314. Sorensen S et al. Dementia care: mental health effects, intervention strategies, and clinical implications. Lancet Neurology, 2006, 5: 961–973.

315. Gallagher-Thompson D, Coon D. Evidence-based psychological treatments for distress in family caregivers of older adults. Psychology and Aging, 2007, 22: 37–51.

316. Hepburn K et al. The Savvy Caregiver program: the demonstrated effectiveness of a transportable dementia caregiver psychoeducation program. Journal of Gerontological Nursing, 2007, 33: 30–36.

317. Burgio L et al. Translating the REACH caregiver intervention for use by area agency on aging personnel: the REACH OUT program. The Gerontologist, 2009, 49: 103–116.

318. Teri L et al. Behavioral treatment of depression in dementia patients: A controlled clinical trial. The Journals of Gerontology. Series B, Psychological sciences and social sciences, 1997, 52: 159–166.

319. Gitlin L et al. Effects of the home environmental skill-building program on the caregiver-care recipient dyad: 6-month outcomes from the Philadelphia REACH Initiative. The Gerontologist, 2003, 43: 532–546.

320. Farran C et al. Psychosocial interventions to reduce depressive symptoms of dementia caregivers: a randomized clinical trial comparing two approaches. Journal of Mental Health and Aging, 2004, 10: 337–350.

321. Gitlin L et al. Maintenance of effects of the home environmental skill-building program for family caregivers and individuals with Alzheimer's disease and related disorders. The Journals of Gerontology. Series A, Biological sciences and medical sciences, 2005, 60: 368–374.

322. Teri L et al. Training community consultants to help family members improve dementia care: a randomized controlled trial. The Gerontologist, 2005, 45: 802–811.

323. Gonyea J, O'Connor M, Boyle P. Project CARE: a randomized controlled trial of a behavioral intervention group for Alzheimer's disease caregivers. The Gerontologist, 2006, 46: 827–832.

324. Gitlin L et al. Tailored activities to manage neuropsychiatric behaviors in persons with dementia and reduce caregiver burden: a randomized pilot study. American Journal of Geriatric Psychiatry, 2008, 16: 229–239.

325. Belle S et al. Enhancing the quality of life of dementia caregivers from different ethnic or racial groups: a randomized, controlled trial. Annals of Internal Medicine, 2006, 145: 727–738.

326. Brodaty H, Gresham M, Luscombe G. The Prince Henry Hospital dementia caregivers' training program. International Journal of Geriatric Psychiatry, 1997, 12: 183–192.

327. Gallagher-Thompson D, Steffen A. Comparative effects of cognitive/behavioral and brief psychodynamic psychotherapies for depressed in family caregivers. Journal of Consulting and Clinical Psychology, 1994, 62 (3): 543–549.

328. Charlesworth GM, Reichelt FK. Keeping conceptualizations simple: examples with family carers of people with dementia. Behavioural and Cognitive Psychotherapy, 2004, 32 (4): 401–409.

329. Knight B, Lutzky S, Macofsky-Urban F. A meta-analytic review of interventions for caregiver distress: recommendations for future research. The Gerontologist, 1993, 33: 240–248.

330. Sorensen S et al. How effective are interventions with caregivers? An updated meta-analysis. The Gerontologist, 2002, 42: 356–372.

331. Woods B. Invited commentary on: Non-pharmacological interventions in dementia. Advances in Psychiatric Treatment, 2010, 10: 178–179.

332. Au A et al. The Coping with Caregiving group program for Chinese caregivers of patients with Alzheimer's disease in Hong Kong. Patient Education and Counseling, 2010, 78: 256–260.

333. Gallagher-Thompson D et al. Families dealing with dementia: insights from mainland China, Hong Kong, and Taiwan. In: Eggleston K, Tuljapurkar S, eds. Aging Asia: economic and social implications of rapid demographic change in China, Japan, and South Korea, 1st ed. Stanford, CA, Shorenstein Asia-Pacific Research Center, 2010.

334. Thompson C et al. Systematic review of information and support interventions for caregivers of people with dementia. BMC Geriatrics, 2007, 7: 18.

335. Magnusson L, Hanson E, Borg M. A literature review study of information and communication technology as a support for frail older people living at home and their family carers. Technology and Disability, 2004, 16: 223–35.

336. Finkel S et al. E-Care: a telecommunications technology intervention for family caregivers of dementia patients. The American Journal of Geriatric Psychiatry: official journal of the American Association for Geriatric Psychiatry, 2007, 15: 443–448.

337. Magnusson L, Hanson E, Nolan M. The impact of information and communication technology on family carers of older people and professionals in Sweden. Ageing and Society, 2005, 25: 693–713.

338. Topo P. Technology studies to meet the needs of people with dementia and their caregivers: a literature review. Journal of Applied Gerontology: the official journal of the Southern Gerontological Society, 2009, 28: 5–37.

339. Lewis M, Hobday J, Hepburn K. Internet-based program for dementia caregivers. American Journal of Alzheimer's Disease and Other Dementias, 2010, 25: 674–679.

340. Chiu T et al. Internet-based caregiver support for Chinese Canadians taking care of a family member with Alzheimer disease and related dementia. Canadian Journal on Aging, 2009, 28: 323–336.

341. Powell J, Chiu T, Eysenbach G. A systematic review of networked technologies supporting carers of people with dementia. Journal of Telemedicine and Telecare, 2008, 14: 154–156.

342. Wortmann M et al. Evolving attitudes to Alzheimer's disease among the general public and caregivers in Europe: findings from the Impact Survey. Journal of Nutrition, Health and Aging, 2010, 14: 531–536.

343. Nielsen-Bohlman L et al. Health literacy: a prescription to end confusion. Washington, DC, The National Academies Press, 2004.

344. Zarcadoolas C, Pleasant A, Greer D. Understanding health literacy: an expanded mode. Health Promotion International, 2005, 20: 195–203.

345. Kwon Y, Kim E. Korean Americans in dementia caregiving research: inclusive strategies to barriers in recruitment. Clinical Gerontologist, 2011, 34: 335–352.

346. Low L-F et al. Future research on dementia relating to culturally and linguistically diverse communities. Australasian Journal on Ageing, 2009, 28 (3): 144–148.

347. Etters L, Goodall D, Harrison B. Caregiver burden among dementia patient caregivers: a review of the literature. The Journal of the American Academy of Nurse Practitioners, 2008, 20: 423–428.

348. Moriarty J, Sharif N, Robinson J. Black and minority ethnic people with dementia and their access to support and services. London, Social Care Institute for Excellence (SCIE), 2011.

349. Carer's strategy and action plan "We care for you". Policy paper. Port Louis, Mauritius, Ministry of Social Security, National Solidarity, Senior Citizens Welfare and Reform Institutions, 2010.

350. Dementia Action Alliance (http://www.dementiaaction.org.uk/info/2/action_plans/4/alzheimers_society, accessed 5 February 2012).

351. Public awareness of dementia: what every commissioner needs to know. London, Alzheimer's Society, 2009.

352. Bond J et al. (2005). Inequalities in dementia care across Europe: key findings of the Facing Dementia Survey. International Journal of Clinical Practice, 59 (Suppl 146): 8–14.

353. Blendon RJ et al. Key findings from a five-country survey of public attitudes about Alzheimer's disease. Poster presented at AAIC, July 2011 (http://www.alzheimer-europe.org/News/Alzheimer-Europe/Wednesday-20-July-2011-International-survey-highlights-great-public-desire-to-seek-early-diagnosis-of-Alzheimer-s, accessed 5 February 2012).

354. Global Alzheimer's fears rise. Alzheimer's Research UK (http://www.alzheimersresearchuk.org/news-detail/10292/Global-Alzheimers-fears-rise/, accessed August 2011).

355. Impact study. London, Alzheimer's Disease International (http://www.alz.co.uk/impact-study, accessed 5 February 2012).

356. National roll-out of the campaign to understand dementia and build community networks (http://www.ninchisho100.net/english/index.html, accessed 5 February 2012).

357. Low L.-F, Anstey KJ. Dementia literacy: recognition and beliefs on dementia of the Australian public. Alzheimer's and Dementia, 2009, 5 (1): 43–49 (http://www.sciencedirect.com/science/article/pii/S1552526008000903, accessed August 2011).

358. Garvey G et al. Making sense of dementia: understanding amongst indigenous Australians. International Journal of Geriatric Psychiatry, 2011, 26 (6): 649–656.

359. US House of Representatives Committee on Foreign Affairs. First congressional hearing on "Global Strategies to Combat the Devastating Health and Economic Impacts of Alzheimer's Disease". Committee News, 24 June 2011 (http://foreignaffairs.house.gov/press_display.asp?id=1879, accessed October 2011).

360. Situational analysis of the management of dementia in Togo. Noncommunicable diseases control office, Ministry of Health Togo. 2011.

361. Quantitative and qualitative research into stigma and dementia. London, The Gate, 2008.

362. Clare L, Goater T, Woods B. Illness representations in early-stage dementia: a preliminary investigation. International Journal of Geriatric Psychiatry, 2006, 21: 761–767.

363. Benbow SM, Reynolds D. Challenging the stigma of Alzheimer's disease. Hospital Medicine, 2000, 61 (3): 174–177.

364. Jolley DJ, Benbow SM. Stigma and Alzheimer's disease: causes, consequences and a constructive approach. International Journal of Clinical Practice, 2000, 54 (2): 117–119.

365. Graham N et al. Reducing stigma and discrimination against older people with mental disorders: a technical consensus statement. International Journal of Geriatric Psychiatry, 2003, 18 (8): 670–678.

366. Dementia. Out of the shadows. London, Alzheimer's Society, 2008.

367. World Alzheimer's Day. Alzheimer's Disease International (http://www.alz.co.uk/world-alzheimers-day, accessed 4 February 2012).

368. Associação Brasileira de Alzheimer (Brazilian Alzheimer Association) (http://www.abraz.com.br/, accessed 8 December 2011).

369. NHS Choices: Dementia. National Health Service in England (http://www.nhs.uk/dementia/, accessed 8 December 2011).

370. Know the 10 signs. Chicago, IL, Alzheimer's Association (http://www.alz.org/alzheimers_disease_know_the_10_signs.asp, accessed, 4 February 2012).

371. Ellena E, Huebner B, eds. I remember better when I paint. Treating Alzheimer's through creative arts (DVD). Paris, French Connection Films (for Hilgos Foundation), 2009.

372. French Connection Film. I remember better when I paint (http://www.youtube.com/watch?v=54AtoQVGfwU, accessed 7 December 2011).

373. Douglas S, James I, Ballard C. Non-pharmacological interventions in dementia. Advances in Psychiatric Treatment, 2004, 10: 171–179.

374. Mind Your Mind. Risk reduction programme of Alzheimer's Australia (http://mindyourmind.org.au/, accessed 4 February 2012).

375. Woodward M et al. Dementia risk reduction: the evidence. Alzheimer's Australia Paper 13. Canberra, Alzheimer's Australia, 2007.

376. Farrow M. Dementia risk reduction: What do Australians know? Alzheimer's Australia Paper 14. Canberra, Alzheimer's Australia, 2008.

377. Towards a national dementia preventative health strategy. Alzheimer's Australia Paper 21. Canberra, Alzheimer's Australia, 2010.

378. New campaign highlighting the devastating impact of Alzheimer's disease. Toronto, Alzheimer Society of Canada, 2010 (http://www.alzheimerbc.org/News-and-Events/News-Archives/2010/Forget-Everything-You-Knew-New.aspx, accessed 6 December 2011).

379. The National Alzheimer's Project Act (NAPA). Chicago, The Alzheimer's Association. (http://www.alz.org/join_the_cause_21243.asp, accessed 4 February 2012).

380. Dementia economic impact report 2008. Alzhemiers New Zealand, 2008 (http://www.alzheimers.org.nz/assets/Reports/AnnualReports/Dementia_Economic_Impact_Report2008.pdf, accessed 11 January 2012).

381. 2011 Alzheimer's disease facts and figures. Alzheimer's Association, 2011 (http://www.alz.org/downloads/Facts_Figures_2011.pdf, accessed 14 September 2011).

382. Creating dementia friendly communities: a guide. Edinburgh, Alzheimer Scotland, 2001.

383. Nicolas Sarkozy, President of the Republic of France. Alzheimer and related diseases plan, 2008 (http://www.plan-alzheimer.gouv.fr/IMG/pdf/discours_PR_France_Sophia_1_fev_2008.pdf, accessed 20 January 2012).

384. Banerjee S, Wittenberg R. Clinical and cost effectiveness of services for early diagnosis and intervention in dementia. International Journal of Geriatric Psychiatry, 2009, 24: 748–754.